Modern Oral Contraception

Updates from
The Contraception Report

Published by
Emron
Totowa, New Jersey
Released June 2000

Emron is a company of IMS Health.

Acknowledgments

The editors wish to thank all the clinicians and writers who have contributed to *The Contraception Report* since its inception. We would also like to thank the staff members at Emron who provided invaluable help in preparing the material for this book. Finally, we acknowledge the ongoing support and commitment of the Women's Health Care Group at Wyeth-Ayerst Laboratories, who generously provided the unrestricted educational grant that made this book possible.

Creative Director: Emily Stetser
Art Director: Kathleen Mercandetti
Administrative Assistant: Diane Haweeny
Editorial Assistant: Joe Simon
Research Coordinator: Phyllis Rossmann
Contributing Writer: Carl Peterson

Library of Congress Catalog Card Number: 00-104259

ISBN: 0-9651745-2-2

First Edition, First Printing

Printed in the United States of America

Table of Contents

Editors

Melinda Wallach, RN
Managing Editor, *The Contraception Report*, Emron—Totowa, New Jersey

David A. Grimes, MD
Vice President of Biomedical Affairs, Family Health International, Research Triangle Park, North Carolina
Clinical Professor, Department of Obstetrics and Gynecology, University of North Carolina School of Medicine—Chapel Hill, North Carolina

Associate Editors

Ernie J. Chaney, MD
Professor Emeritus, Department of Family and Community Medicine, The University of Kansas School of Medicine, Wichita — Wichita, Kansas

Elizabeth B. Connell, MD
Professor Emeritus, Department of Gynecology and Obstetrics, Emory University School of Medicine—Atlanta, Georgia

Mitchell D. Creinin, MD
Associate Professor, Department of Obstetrics, Gynecology, and Reproductive Sciences, Magee-Womens Hospital, University of Pittsburgh School of Medicine—Pittsburgh, Pennsylvania

S. Jean Emans, MD
Chief, Division of Adolescent/Young Adult Medicine, Children's Hospital
Associate Professor of Pediatrics, Harvard Medical School—Boston, Massachusetts

Joseph W. Goldzieher, MD
Distinguished Professor, Department of Obstetrics and Gynecology, Texas Tech University Health Sciences Center—Amarillo, Texas

Paula J. A. Hillard, MD
Professor, Departments of Obstetrics & Gynecology and Pediatrics, University of Cincinnati College of Medicine—Cincinnati, Ohio

Luigi Mastroianni, Jr., MD
William Goodell Professor of Obstetrics and Gynecology, University of Pennsylvania Medical Center—Philadelphia, Pennsylvania

Preface

Modern Oral Contraception provides clinicians with a user-friendly handbook covering a wide variety of topics related to this method of birth control. We have tried to rely upon science and not our collective experience or opinions. The text contains four sections, each of which is divided into subsections. Each subsection summarizes the best available evidence on the topic and contains *Take Home Messages* that give the reader key points in an abbreviated, easy-to-read style. While the editors have reviewed hundreds of publications in the preparation of this book, references in each section are generally limited to those that are current and most pertinent.

The terms *oral contraceptives* and *OCs* are used interchangeably. Unless otherwise noted, these terms refer to combination oral contraceptives containing estrogen and progestin. Discussion of progestin-only OCs appears separately in Section 4.4. For ease of reading, common terms are abbreviated at first mention and used interchangeably thereafter. Some less common terms are abbreviated each time they appear. Readers can find a complete list of abbreviations in Appendix C.

We focus on the clinical aspects of prescribing, including those that have been the subject of controversy or misinformation. For example, we present various perspectives on the debate concerning OCs and venous thromboembolism and examine whether screening for thrombophilic abnormalities is cost-effective. In addition, we explore whether OC progestins are "androgenic," whether women with sickle cell anemia can use OCs, and how the media have influenced women's perceptions of OCs.

Oral contraception offers women the opportunity to control their fertility, improve their health, and contribute to the well-being of their families. Serious complications of birth control pills are infrequent. We hope you find this information useful in your practice and welcome your feedback.

Sincerely yours,

Melinda Wallach, RN
Editor

David A. Grimes, MD
Editor

Note to Readers: Interpretation of Risk

Throughout this book, the editors use several terms that measure risk. These terms include relative risk, odds ratio, and confidence interval. For those unfamiliar with these concepts, the following brief explanation and sample graphic should help interpretation of various study data reported in this book.

A relative risk (RR) is a measure of association that can be obtained from prospective studies. An RR of 1.0 indicates no association between the exposure (eg, oral contraceptives) and the outcome (eg, stroke). A relative risk greater than 1.0 indicates an increased risk; an RR lower than 1.0 indicates a decreased risk. An odds ratio (OR) is a measure of association derived from case-control studies and is a good approximation of relative risk for infrequent diseases.

A relative risk must be interpreted in light of its confidence interval (CI). Confidence intervals indicate how precise the RR estimate is. A narrow confidence interval implies good precision and vice versa. Confidence intervals that exclude 1.0 are considered statistically significant at the p<0.05 level.

Examples of Relative Risks with 95% Confidence Intervals

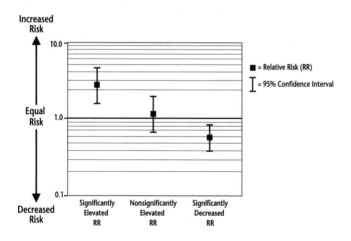

Continuing Medical Education Accreditation

Statement of Need: Clinicians need to stay informed about the most up-to-date findings concerning oral contraception. Clinicians involved in reproductive health care need to understand the evolution and ongoing development of oral contraceptives. They also need to have current data concerning the efficacy, safety, and side effect profile of modern, low-dose OCs. In addition, clinicians need information concerning ways to encourage successful use of OCs.

Goal: The broad mission of the Editorial Board for *The Contraception Report* is to develop patient education and professional communication materials that address the benefits and risks of contraceptives, as well as other reproductive health-related issues, in a scientifically balanced manner.

Educational Objectives:

After reading Section 1 of this book, participants will be able to:

1) state the reason why lower steroid doses in combination birth control pills still maintain contraceptive efficacy;
2) identify the proportion of retail OC prescriptions written for low-dose pills (≤35 µg ethinyl estradiol) in 1998;
3) state the trend in use of oral contraceptives among women aged 35 years and older between 1982 and 1995;
4) identify one reason why the World Health Organization (WHO) and other international organizations decided to reevaluate the evidence concerning medical eligibility criteria for oral contraceptives; and,
5) explain the metabolic effects of combination OCs that produce a beneficial effect on acne.

After reading Section 2 of this book, participants will be able to:

6) state the approximate risk of ischemic and hemorrhagic stroke found in women taking low-dose OCs in the Kaiser Permanente health maintenance organization in the United States;
7) state the finding of WHO and the Royal College of General Practitioners regarding the risk of myocardial infarction among nonsmoking women taking OCs;

8) identify two main findings of the Collaborative Group on Hormonal Factors in Breast Cancer with regard to use of oral contraceptives and breast cancer;

9) state the approximate risk of gallbladder disease found with OC use from the 1994 analysis of the Oxford Family Planning Association Study; and,

10) describe the World Health Organization's recommendations for using combination OCs in women with sickle cell anemia and sickle cell trait.

After reading Section 3 of this book, participants will be able to:

11) state one health benefit of the pill that may help to improve consistent OC use among teens;

12) state the Food and Drug Administration's position regarding off-label use of drugs;

13) identify at least three noncontraceptive medical uses of combined OCs;

14) identify two fears women often have concerning oral contraceptives; and,

15) state the proportion of OC discontinuers (1995 National Survey of Family Growth data) who are using no method of contraception 3 months later.

After reading Section 4 of this book, participants will be able to:

16) describe the association between hormonal contraception use and HIV susceptibility;

17) identify the proportion of pregnancies prevented by progestin-only emergency contraceptive pills;

18) describe the latest findings concerning the effectiveness and side effect profile for levonorgestrel used alone for emergency contraception;

19) state the estimated first-year typical use failure rate for progestin-only OCs; and,

20) identify the length of time progestin-only OC users should use backup contraception in the event of late or missed pills.

Educational Method: The information is presented in monograph format as four separate sections. It should take the reader 8 hours to complete all four sections (2 hours to complete each section). Each section consists of several subsections, a post-test and an evaluation form. Participants should, in order, read the Preface, Interpretation of Risk, and Continuing Medical Accreditation (includes the learning objectives). The participant should then read a section, complete the post-test and complete the quiz answer form for the section read. To obtain CME credit for the section, follow the instructions found on the CME Quiz Answer Form. CME certificates will be issued for each section (up to 2 hours of AMA Physician's Recognition Award category 1 credit per section). Expiration date for CME credit is June 30, 2001.

Evaluation: Four evaluation forms provide readers with the opportunity to review the content of the book, to identify future educational needs, and to comment on any perceived commercial or promotional bias in the presentation.

Evaluation Instrument: Four 10-question, multiple-choice CME quizzes are used as the evaluation instruments.

Intended or Target Audience: This book is intended for obstetricians and gynecologists, family physicians, pediatricians, adolescent medicine specialists, nurse practitioners, nurse midwives, and others involved in reproductive health care.

CME Information: This activity has been planned and implemented in accordance with the Essential Areas and Policies of the Accreditation Council for Continuing Medical Education (ACCME) through the joint sponsorship of the Dannemiller Memorial Educational Foundation and Emron. The Dannemiller Memorial Educational Foundation is accredited by the ACCME to provide continuing medical education for physicians.

The Dannemiller Memorial Educational Foundation designates this educational activity for up to 8 hours in Category 1 credit toward the AMA Physician's Recognition Award. Each physician should claim only those hours of credit that he/she actually spent in the educational activity.

Provider approved by the California Board of Registered Nursing, Provider Number 4229 for 8 contact hours.

Disclosure Information

The Dannemiller Memorial Educational Foundation requires that the faculty participating in a continuing medical education activity disclose to participants any significant financial interest or other relationship (1) with the manufacturer(s) of any commercial product(s) and/or provider(s) of commercial services discussed in an educational presentation, and (2) with any commercial supporters of the activity.

David A. Grimes, MD, has performed research supported by Berlex, Ortho, and Wyeth-Ayerst. He has been a consultant for ALZA, GynoPharma, Mead Johnson, Ortho, Schmid, Searle, Schering, Organon, and Gynétics. He has served on the speakers' bureaus of Berlex, GynoPharma, Ortho, Parke-Davis, and Wyeth-Ayerst.

Ernie J. Chaney, MD, has no relationship that impacts on this activity.

Elizabeth B. Connell, MD, has no relationship that impacts on this activity.

Mitchell D. Creinin, MD, has performed research for Ortho, Organon, and Wyeth-Ayerst. He serves as a consultant for Berlex. He has received honoraria from Ortho, Wyeth-Ayerst, and Pharmacia & Upjohn.

S. Jean Emans, MD, has received research grants and honoraria from Upjohn, Wyeth-Ayerst, Ortho, Syntex, and Pfizer.

Joseph W. Goldzieher, MD, has no relationship that impacts on this activity.

Paula J. A. Hillard, MD, is a consultant for, and has received research grants from, Proctor & Gamble. She serves on the speakers' bureaus of Wyeth-Ayerst, Berlex, Parke-Davis, and Pharmacia & Upjohn.

Luigi Mastroianni, Jr., MD, is a sponsored speaker of Organon, Wyeth-Ayerst, and Searle.

1.1: History and Development

Key scientific discoveries, a wealthy widow, and a dose of serendipity all played a role in the development of the combination oral contraceptive. Furthermore, within this story lies the explanation of why birth control pills have evolved into the low-dose formulations available today.

Two key discoveries regarding progesterone made oral contraceptives (OCs) possible.[1] In the early 1940s, chemist Russell E. Marker found an economical way to produce progesterone from a Mexican plant, *Dioscorea mexicana*. In the early 1950s, Carl Djerassi and Frank Colton, both chemists, independently discovered how to make orally active progestins, a crucial advance because progesterone has negligible oral potency.

Synthetic estrogens were first developed in the early 1930s, when researchers isolated crystalline estrone and then discovered how to convert it to estradiol.[2] In 1938, a far more potent version of estradiol, ethinyl estradiol (EE), was synthesized. Physicians used the hormone to treat various gynecological disorders, including dysmenorrhea. Several scientists had noted the ovulation-inhibiting properties of estrogen early on, even suggesting its use as "hormonal sterilization."

In 1950, a wealthy widow, Katherine McCormick, sought to use her fortune to support the birth control movement. She and Margaret Sanger, the famed visiting nurse who championed birth control earlier in the century, approached several scientists, including Gregory Pincus, a Harvard physiologist and leading authority on reproductive biology and the mammalian egg. Pincus recruited Min-Chueh Chang, a reproductive biologist, and John Rock, MD, a Professor of Gynecology at Harvard Medical School.

These scientists were working with the progestational agents norethynodrel and norethindrone to develop a progestin-only oral contraceptive. They decided upon the original dose of 10 mg of norethynodrel after extrapolation from animal data. Importantly, however, the norethynodrel coming from the factory was contaminated with 0.15% of an estrogen, mestranol. To a chemist, 0.15% contamination is minute; however, in pills containing 10 mg of norethynodrel, that small percentage translated into the relatively large dose of 150 µg mestranol.

The importance of mestranol was recognized when the norethynodrel coming from the factory became purer. As the mestranol was eliminated, the pill provided less effective cycle control. The researchers then decided to keep the estrogen in the formulation for its beneficial effect on cycle control.

No one recognized, however, that the mestranol also had powerful contraceptive effects. At that time, it was known that estrogens of other kinds—conjugated equine estrogens, estradiol, and others—do not inhibit the pituitary very well. However, the 17 α-ethinyl group, which is present in mestranol and ethinyl estradiol, confers an extraordinary amount of pituitary-inhibiting action, a property not shared by any other type of derivative.[3]

This unique contraceptive property prompted further investigation into various oral contraceptive preparations. Research on pills with lower estrogen doses showed that the estrogen and progestin acted *synergistically* to inhibit the pituitary. Therefore, it required even less of each component for effective ovulation inhibition than might have been anticipated from their individual effects. This finding was the breakthrough that made possible the current generation of low-dose OCs containing ≤35 µg ethinyl estrogen.

References

1. Perone N. The progestins. In: Goldzieher JW, Fotherby K, eds. *Pharmacology of the Contraceptive Steroids*. New York: Raven Press; 1994:5-19.

2. Goldzieher JW. The estrogens. In: Goldzieher JW, Fotherby K, eds. *Pharmacology of the Contraceptive Steroids*. New York: Raven Press; 1994:21-25.

3. Goldzieher JW, de la Pena A, Chenault CB. Ovulation inhibiting action of ethynyl estrogen. *Fertil Steril* 1974;25:299-300.

1.2: Trends in OC Use

The National Survey of Family Growth (NSFG) is a large, national survey of US women of reproductive age conducted by the National Center for Health Statistics of the Centers for Disease Control and Prevention (CDC). According to the 1995 NSFG, oral contraceptive use has declined among many populations, including younger women and those never married. On the other hand, OC use has more than doubled among women aged 35 to 39 years.[1]

The 1995 NSFG found that more women used contraception in 1995 than in 1982 or 1987. Female sterilization alone (not including male sterilization) became the most popular method of contraception, followed by oral contraceptives and the male condom. The number of contraceptive users among women aged 15 to 44 years increased from about 30 million in 1982 to nearly 39 million in 1995. Approximately 64% of reproductive age women were practicing contraception in 1995 compared to 56% in 1982.

Overall, the distribution of contraceptive users by method remained relatively steady between 1988 and 1995 (Figure 1). Between 1982 and 1995, however, substantial changes occurred in OC use. Overall pill use among women declined from 31% in 1982 to 27% in 1995. The largest decreases occurred among black women younger than age 25 years. Among teenage black women, use of the pill dropped by almost 60% between 1988 and 1995—from 75% to 32%. Among black women aged 20 to 24 years, pill use declined by 36%. Why young black women stopped using the pill is not known; however, 5% used implants and 8% used injectable contraception. In addition, dramatic increases (sixfold) in male condom use occurred among this population, presumably due to human immunodeficiency virus/acquired immunodeficiency syndrome (HIV/AIDS) education campaigns.

The decline in OC use was also greater among women in their teens and early 20s than among older women. Between 1988 and 1995, the percentage of contracepting teenagers using the pill fell from 59% to 44%; among women aged 20 to 24 years, the percentage dropped from 68% to 52% (Figure 2). The decline in pill use accompanied an increase in male condom use among teens.

Figure 1

Percentage of Women Aged 15 to 44 Years Using Contraception by Current Method—NSFG* 1982, 1988, and 1995

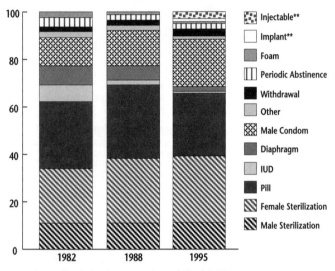

*National Survey of Family Growth   **Data available only in 1995

Source: Piccinino LJ and Mosher WD, 1998 (see reference 1).

Among women aged 30 years and over, on the other hand, OC use increased. Between 1982 and 1995, pill use among women aged 35 to 39 years doubled and increased sixfold among those aged 40 to 44 years. The increase in pill use among older women may be due, in part, to the increased recognition that healthy, nonsmoking women can safely take OCs until menopause and that use of OCs confers a number of well-documented health benefits, including relief of perimenopausal symptoms, protection against ovarian and endometrial cancers, and prevention of ectopic pregnancy.

Trends in OC use also varied by race/ethnicity. For example, little change occurred in the proportion of white women using OCs between 1988 and 1995. On the other hand, pill use declined substantially among Hispanic women, from 33% to 23%, and among black women, from 38% to 24%.

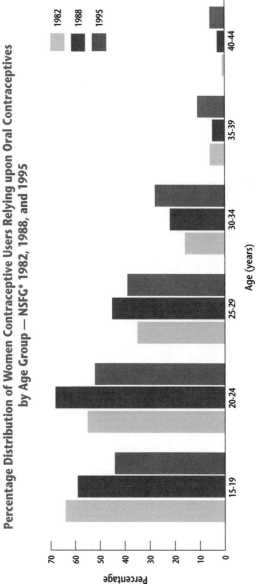

Figure 2

Percentage Distribution of Women Contraceptive Users Relying upon Oral Contraceptives by Age Group — NSFG* 1982, 1988, and 1995

*National Survey of Family Growth

Source: Piccinino LJ and Mosher WD, 1998 (see reference 1).

Dual Method Use

The growing threat of HIV and other sexually transmitted diseases (STDs) has led to an increased interest in the role of dual contraceptive use. Nevertheless, in 1995, only 9% of contraceptive users reported that they used more than one method. Of those who used multiple methods, virtually all used the male condom as one of their choices.

The most common combinations were condoms with OCs (used by about a third of multiple-method users), condoms with withdrawal (used by about a quarter), and condoms with the calendar rhythm method (used by about 17%). Women younger than 25 years who were single and college educated were more likely to report using dual methods than other women.

Dual method use varied by age. Teenagers (8%) were most likely to rely upon condoms with the pill and condoms with withdrawal, while fewer than 1% of women aged 40 to 44 years did so. Despite efforts to encourage dual method use, most women still rely primarily upon one method. Women using OCs need to be encouraged to use male latex condoms if they are at risk of STDs.

Take Home Messages

- *Between 1982 and 1995, OC use declined and male condom use increased*
- *Pill use declined among younger women and increased among women aged 30 years and older*
- *Despite the risk of HIV and other STDs, few women used dual methods*

Reference

1. Piccinino LJ, Mosher WD. Trends in contraceptive use in the United States: 1982-1995. *Fam Plann Perspect* 1998;30:4-10,46.

1.3: Trends in OC Prescribing

Oral contraceptives have changed substantially since their introduction in the early 1960s. Early formulations contained much higher levels of estrogen and progestin than today's low-dose pills. This change came about after researchers discovered that the estrogen and progestin components of combined OCs act synergistically to inhibit the pituitary, requiring less of each for ovulation inhibition. As manufacturers have developed lower-dose pills, prescribing patterns have also changed.

A 1991 analysis of prescribing trends reported a dramatic decrease in the percentage of OC prescriptions written for pills containing ≥50 μg estrogen between 1968 and 1988. In 1968, more than 99% of all retail OC prescriptions were for formulations containing ≥50 μg of estrogen. Twenty years later, this number had fallen to 18% (Figure 3).[1]

The *National Prescription Audit* of IMS HEALTH (Plymouth Meeting, Pennsylvania) tracks the number of prescriptions dispensed by retail pharmacies in the contiguous United States. These data were used by the editors of *The Contraception Report* to

Figure 3

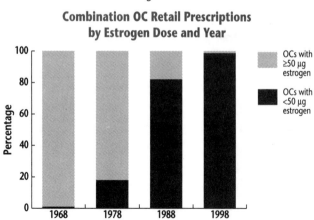

Combination OC Retail Prescriptions by Estrogen Dose and Year

Source: Gerstman BB, et al, 1991 (see reference 1) and IMS HEALTH, National Prescription Audit, November 1998.

evaluate trends in low-dose (<50 µg estrogen) oral contraceptive use. Data for 1998 indicate that 50 µg estrogen pills account for fewer than 1 million of the 68.5 million annual OC prescriptions—approximately 1.4% (Figure 4).

30 and 35 µg Estrogen Formulations

The overall number of OC prescriptions rose 10% between 1996 and 1998. In 1998, roughly 30 million prescriptions were written for 30 µg pills; just over 32 million 35 µg OC prescriptions were dispensed that same year. Together, these two OC formulations account for more than 90% of the OC market.

After rising by more than 30% between 1991 and 1996, the number of monophasic OC prescriptions leveled off in recent years, growing less than 4% between 1996 and 1998. Meanwhile, the number of multiphasic OCs dispensed over the 2-year period grew by more than 20%.

Monophasic OC preparations now account for 58% of the OC market (Figure 5). Among multiphasic pills, triphasics account for nearly all prescriptions dispensed. Biphasic pills are rarely prescribed (0.1% of all OC prescriptions in 1998).

Figure 4

Percentage of Retail Prescriptions Written for Oral Contraceptives by Estrogen Dose—1998

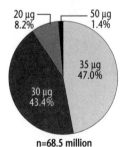

n=68.5 million

Source: IMS HEALTH, National Prescription Audit, *November 1998.*

Figure 5

Percentage of Retail Prescriptions Written for Low-Dose* Oral Contraceptives by Progestin Phasing—1998

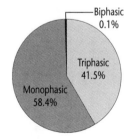

*Oral contraceptives containing <50 µg estrogen

Source: IMS HEALTH, National Prescription Audit, *November 1998.*

Use of 20 μg Estrogen Formulations

Use of 20 μg pills has increased over the past decade. During the first half of the decade, the number of prescriptions for 20 μg OCs (one product, which became available in the mid-1970s) increased 10-fold. This trend has continued since 1997, as three additional monophasic 20 μg products were introduced.

In 1996, 20 μg pills accounted for just under 4% of all OC prescriptions. By 1998, that number had more than doubled to 8.2%. The total number of 20 μg prescriptions rose 143% over the 2-year period, from 2.3 million in 1996 to 5.6 million in 1998.

The past several years have also seen a marked decrease in the age of patients using 20 μg pills. In 1996, women aged 40 years and older accounted for nearly half of all 20 μg pill prescriptions. By 1998, this number had dropped to about 28% (Figure 6). Women aged 20 to 39 years now use nearly 60% of all 20 μg pills prescribed, up from 44% 2 years ago. The proportion of adolescents and teens using 20 μg preparations has doubled since 1996, as well.

Whether these trends in OC prescribing will continue is unknown. Furthermore, the data do not provide insight into the cause(s) or importance, if any, of these prescribing patterns. These changes may be due to promotion of products and do not necessarily reflect a scientific rationale for changes in product prescribing.

Methodology

The editors separated prescriptions containing 20, 30, and 35 μg estrogen. Pills containing 50 μg mestranol were grouped with 35 μg estrogen pills. Mestranol must be converted to the active estrogen, ethinyl estradiol. Data indicate that 30% of mestranol is lost in this conversion, making 50 μg mestranol pills bioequivalent to 35 μg EE formulations.[2]

We also looked at trends in use of monophasic or multiphasic preparations, again limiting the analysis to low-dose formulations. We included multiphasic pills with consistent use of 35 μg EE throughout the cycle with 35 μg estrogen products. Those multiphasic pills using less than a mean of 35 μg of estrogen were included with 30 μg products. Doing so did not change the trend for 30 μg pills.

Age data were derived from the *National Disease and Therapeutic Index*, IMS HEALTH, which tracks data from US office-based physicians.

Figure 6

Age of Women Using Oral Contraceptives with 20 µg Estrogen, 1996 and 1998

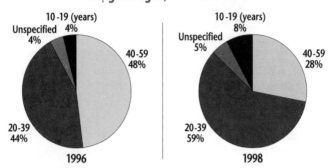

Source: IMS HEALTH, National Disease and Therapeutic Index, November 1998.

Take Home Messages

- Nearly all OC prescriptions today are for pills containing ≤35 µg estrogen

- Clinicians increasingly are prescribing multiphasic preparations, up more than 20% in 2 years

- The number of prescriptions for monophasic 20 µg OCs more than doubled between 1996 and 1998 as several new products entered the market

- These lowest-dose pills are also being used by younger patients

---

References

1. Gerstman BB, Gross TP, Kennedy DL, et al. Trends in the content and use of oral contraceptives in the United States, 1964-1988. *Am J Public Health* 1991; 81:90-98.

2. Brody SA, Turkes A, Goldzieher JW. Pharmacokinetics of three bioequivalent norethindrone/mestranol-50 µg and three norethindrone/ethinyl estradiol-35 µg OC formulations. Are "low-dose" pills really lower? *Contraception* 1989;40:269-284.

1.4: Mechanisms of Action/Efficacy

Modern low-dose oral contraceptives (containing 20 to 35 µg of estrogen) are possible because of the potent contraceptive effects of both ethinyl estrogens and synthetic progestins.

Almost all of today's low-dose oral contraceptives contain the estrogen ethinyl estradiol, although a few contain mestranol (the methyl ether of ethinyl estradiol). Mestranol must be converted to the active estrogen, ethinyl estradiol. Data indicate that 30% of mestranol is lost in the conversion, making 50 µg mestranol pills bioequivalent to 35 µg EE formulations.[1,2]

Several concepts are essential to understand the properties of estrogens used in today's low-dose OCs:

- Ethinyl estrogens profoundly suppress gonadotropin secretion by the pituitary and, consequently, prevent ovulation; and,

- Ethinyl estrogens work *synergistically* with synthetic progestins. Thus, very little of each hormone is necessary to produce a contraceptive effect.

When taken orally, ethinyl estrogens are absorbed from the stomach and sulfated rapidly by the liver; that which is excreted in the bile is, to some extent, deconjugated in the intestine. These effects (enterohepatic recirculation) account for the large first-pass metabolism (40% to 60%).[2]

Importantly, metabolism by the liver and gut results in large variations in bioavailability. Consequently, a very large intra- and interindividual variability exists in metabolism of EE among women. Plasma EE levels after OC ingestion vary substantially from woman to woman. Furthermore, the same woman may process and metabolize EE differently from day to day. Other factors that impact the metabolism of EE include ethnicity, body weight, and nutritional status. These intra- and interindividual variations in metabolism of EE make it difficult, if not impossible, to predict with any certainty how a woman will respond to a particular OC.

Synthetic progestins used in OCs available in the US today include estranes and gonanes. Orally active progestins are absorbed rapidly from the upper gastrointestinal tract and bioavailability varies depending upon the progestin.

Table 1

Mechanisms of Action of Combination OCs

Confirmed

- *Suppression of ovulation via hypothalamic and pituitary effects*
  - *Diminished frequency of gonadotropin-releasing hormone (GnRH) pulses*
  - *Decreased pituitary responsiveness to GnRH*
  - *Suppression of luteinizing and follicle-stimulating hormones*
  - *Absence of luteinizing hormone surge*
- *Progestin-mediated alterations in the consistency and properties of cervical mucus*

Unconfirmed

- *Alterations in the endometrial lining*
- *Alterations of tubal transport mechanisms*

Estrogens exert their contraceptive effect primarily by suppressing luteinizing and follicle-stimulating hormones (LH and FSH) and preventing ovulation (Table 1). Progestins also suppress these two gonadotropins.

Other mechanisms of action likely support the efficacy of combination OCs.[2,3] For example, the progestational agent makes the cervical mucus more viscous, scanty, and cellular. These effects are thought to impede the ascent of both sperm and organisms into the upper reproductive tract, helping to protect OC users from pregnancy and some nonviral STDs. Other possible, but unconfirmed, mechanisms of action include alterations in the endometrium and tubal transport processes.

Efficacy

Combination oral contraceptives are highly effective at preventing pregnancy when they are used consistently and correctly (perfect use). During perfect use, failure rates are estimated to be <1%. Because OCs require daily user compliance, however, typical failure rates (which take into account variations in consistency of use) are higher. Analysis of data from the 1995 National Survey of Family Growth, which includes correction for abortion underreporting, indicates that the average OC user experiences a typical failure rate of 4% during the first 6 months of use and 7% during the first 12 months of use.[4]

In fact, most pill failures are due to user mistakes, rather than method failure. The critical factor in efficacy is not "theoretical effectiveness," but user compliance. Compliance is intimately related to side effects and the user's perceptions of risks and benefits, a factor heavily influenced by media-generated misinformation. (For further discussion, see the sections on the media's impact on perceptions regarding the birth control pill and successful OC use.)

Should efficacy be a concern when using very low-dose (20 µg) pills? The data are reassuring that low-dose pills are effective. The clinical trials of pills with 20 µg EE show the pregnancy rate is no different than with 35 µg pills.

Two reports suggested that lower-dose OCs were associated with higher failure rates. One, a retrospective investigation by Meade et al, found about twice as much risk of failure with lower-dose formulations (30 µg EE).[5] In practical reality, however, the chance of failure was so small as to be inconsequential. The 50 µg and 30 µg preparations had failure rates between 0.1 and 0.2 per 100 woman-years.

The other study, by Ketting, utilized data recorded from women obtaining an abortion in the Netherlands from 1982 to 1984.[6] In the Netherlands, over 1 million women use OCs. From detailed interviews, Ketting estimated that the true OC failure rate (ie, with correct use) was an extraordinary 0.02 pregnancies per 100 woman-years for all types of OCs combined. The pregnancy rates were no different for monophasic OCs containing 50 µg EE compared to those with <50 µg EE.

Take Home Messages

- *Ethinyl estrogens work synergistically with synthetic progestins to inhibit ovulation*
- *Progestational effects on the cervical mucus also enhance contraceptive efficacy*
- *The typical failure rate for OCs is about 7% in the first 12 months of use*
- *If taken correctly and consistently, however, the OC failure rate is estimated to be <1%*

References

1.   Brody SA, Turkes A, Goldzieher JW. Pharmacokinetics of three bioequivalent norethindrone/mestranol-50 µg and three norethindrone/ethinyl estradiol-35 µg OC formulations. Are "low-dose" pills really lower? *Contraception* 1989;40:269-284.

2.   Goldzieher JW. *Hormonal Contraception: Pills, Injections & Implants*. 4th ed. Ontario: EMIS-CANADA; 1998.

3.   Hardman JG, Limbird LE, eds. *Goodman & Gilman's The Pharmacological Basis of Therapeutics*. 9th ed. Section XIII: Hormones and hormone synthesis. New York: The McGraw-Hill Companies, Inc.; 1996.

4.   Fu H, Darroch JE, Haas T, et al. Contraceptive failure rates: new estimates from the 1995 National Survey of Family Growth. *Fam Plann Perspect* 1999;31:58-63.

5.   Meade TW, Greenberg G, Thompson SG. Progestogens and cardiovascular reactions associated with oral contraceptives and a comparison of the safety of 50- and 30-microgram oestrogen preparations. *BMJ* 1980;280:1157-1161.

6.   Ketting E. The relative reliability of oral contraceptives; findings of an epi-demiological study. *Contraception* 1988;37:343-348.

1.5: OC Progestins

The estrogen component of oral contraceptives is relatively uniform across all OC formulations. Consequently, progestins in oral contraceptives have been the focus of intense scrutiny over the past decade.

i. Classification

Norethindrone and levonorgestrel belong to two distinct classes of synthetic progestins. Norethindrone and other progestins that metabolize to norethindrone are estranes. Levonorgestrel and related compounds are gonanes. Estranes and gonanes exhibit different metabolic characteristics.

The terminology used to classify OC progestins has become confusing because terms such as "new," "newer," "second generation," and "third generation" have been used under no standard guidelines.[1,2] Progestins often have been grouped together improperly in categories based on time since market introduction, rather than by pharmacological properties. The "second-generation" category often groups levonorgestrel- and norethindrone-containing products together, while the "third-generation" category often includes the progestins gestodene (not available in the United States) and desogestrel. To add to the confusion, norgestimate, which metabolizes primarily to levonorgestrel, has been labeled "second generation"; however, others have considered this progestin a "third-generation" product because of its market introduction (in Europe) around the same time as desogestrel and gestodene.

Lumping levonorgestrel and norethindrone together ignores both the structure and basic pharmacology of the drugs.[3-5] Norethindrone and those compounds that metabolize to norethindrone are estranes. Progestins of this type available in the US include norethindrone, norethindrone acetate, and ethynodiol diacetate. These synthetic estranes convert to the biologically active component norethindrone (Table 2).

Levonorgestrel and its "cousins" are gonane progestins. The gonanes include norgestrel (specifically, its levo-enantiomer *levonorgestrel*, which is biologically active), desogestrel, gestodene, and norgestimate. Each of these progestins has a different biologically

Table 2

Classification of Progestins Used in Oral Contraceptives

19-Nortestosterone (parent hormone)	Biologically Active Compound(s)
Estranes	
Ethynodiol Diacetate	Norethindrone
Lynestrenol*	Norethindrone
Norethindrone	Norethindrone
Norethindrone acetate	Norethindrone
Norethynodrel*	Norethindrone
Gonanes	
Desogestrel	3-keto-desogestrel
Gestodene*	Gestodene
Levonorgestrel	Levonorgestrel
Norgestimate	Levonorgestrel Levonorgestrel-3-oxime

*Not available in US
Sources: Adapted from references 3-5.

active component, although it appears that norgestimate is largely metabolized to levonorgestrel.

The terms "second-" and "third-generation" progestins, as used today, are misleading. Grouping estrane and gonane progestins together is similar to lumping separate classes of antihypertensives together. For example, clinicians would not group calcium channel blockers and beta-blockers together in a research study and presume they have the same effects. Calcium channel blockers and beta-blockers have distinct and unique mechanisms of action, pharmacological properties, and side-effect profiles. Grouping gonanes and estranes together is likewise inappropriate.

Gonane and estrane progestins differ substantially.[3-5] The drugs have different serum half-lives and bioavailability. A listing of branded low-dose OCs on the US market (and generic equivalents) containing either estrane or gonane progestins can be helpful to identify clearly which products contain which type of progestin (Tables 3 and 4).

Table 3	*Table 4*
US Low-Dose Combination OC Products Containing Estrane Progestins	**US Low-Dose Combination OC Products Containing Gonane Progestins**

Ethynodiol Diacetate
Demulen 1/35†

Norethindrone
Modicon, Brevicon††
Ortho-Novum 10/11, Jenest*
Ortho-Novum 1/35, Norinyl 1/35**
Ortho-Novum 7/7/7
Ovcon-35
Tri-Norinyl

Norethindrone Acetate
Estrostep
Loestrin 1/20
Loestrin 1.5/30

† *Generic equivalent includes Zovia 1/35*

†† *Generic equivalents include Necon 0.5/35, Nelova 0.5/35*

* *Generic equivalents include Necon 10/11, Nelova 10/11*

** *Generic equivalents include Necon 1/35, Nelova 1/35*

Desogestrel
Mircette
Ortho-Cept, Desogen

Norgestrel/Levonorgestrel
Alesse, Levlite
Lo/Ovral*
Nordette, Levlen†
Triphasil, Tri-Levlen**

Norgestimate
Ortho-Cyclen
Ortho Tri-Cyclen

* *Generic equivalent includes Low-Ogestrel*
† *Generic equivalent includes Levora*
** *Generic equivalent includes Trivora*

Brand names are for identification purposes only and do not imply endorsement.

Take Home Messages

- *The terms "new," "newer," "second generation" and "third generation" do not accurately describe OC progestins*
- *Norethindrone and those compounds that metabolize to norethindrone are estranes*
- *Levonorgestrel and related progestins (desogestrel, gestodene, and norgestimate) are gonane progestins*

References

1. Carr BR. Uniqueness of oral contraceptive progestins. *Contraception* 1998; 58(suppl):23S-27S.

2. Hannaford P. The collection and interpretation of epidemiological data about the cardiovascular risks associated with the use of steroid contraceptives. *Contraception* 1998;57:137-142.

3. Stanczyk FZ, Roy S. Metabolism of levonorgestrel, norethindrone, and structurally related contraceptive steroids. *Contraception* 1990;42:67-96.

4. Stanczyk FZ. Pharmacokinetics of the new progestogens and influence of gestodene and desogestrel on ethinylestradiol metabolism. *Contraception* 1997;55:273-282.

5. Fotherby K. Pharmacokinetics and metabolism of progestins in humans. In: Goldzieher JW, Fotherby K, eds. *Pharmacology of the Contraceptive Steroids*. New York: Raven Press; 1994:99-126.

ii. Pharmacokinetics

Three main pharmacological considerations for contraceptive progestins are bioavailability, serum half-life, and relative binding affinity (RBA). These pharmacokinetic properties affect required dosages, cycle control, and contraceptive protection in the event of missed pills.

The key function of progestins in combined oral contraceptives (in synergy with the ethinyl estrogen) is to inhibit ovulation by suppressing gonadotropin release. All available OC progestins do this, but not all follow the same pharmacokinetic path. Understanding the pharmacokinetic variations among OC progestins may be useful when prescribing pills. OC progestins differ in three key areas: bioavailability (due to hepatic transformation), serum half-life, and relative binding affinity (Table 5).[1-11]

Bioavailability and Hepatic Transformation

The bioavailability of contraceptive progestins reflects the extent to which they are metabolized by the liver during "first-pass" metabolism. As a rule, higher bioavailability is desirable for OC progestins, reducing the oral dose required and resulting in less patient-to-patient variation.[1]

The bioavailability of OC progestins varies considerably, in part because some must be transformed into biologically active forms before taking effect. Progestins that must undergo such transformation are often referred to as "prodrugs" or "prohormones." They include norethindrone acetate and ethynodiol diacetate (which are

Table 5

Posthepatic Bioavailability, Serum Half-Life, and Relative Binding Affinity for Human Uterine Progesterone Receptor for Progestins in Combined Oral Contraceptives

OC Progestin	Bioavailability	Serum Half-Life	Relative Binding Affinity (Human)**
Desogestrel 3-keto-desogestrel	62%	12 hours	180%
Gestodene*	≥90%	12 hours	70%
Levonorgestrel	90%	15 hours	250%
Norethindrone	64%	7 hours	130%
Norgestimate			
Levonorgestrel	22%	15 hours	250%
Levonorgestrel-17-acetate	?	?	110%
Levonorgestrel-3-oxime	?	?	8%

*Not available in the US
**As compared with reference compound R5020

Sources: Adapted from references 2-5, 7, and 10.

metabolized to norethindrone), desogestrel (which is converted to 3-keto-desogestrel), and norgestimate (which is metabolized into levonorgestrel, levonorgestrel-17-acetate, and levonorgestrel-3-oxime). Norethindrone, levonorgestrel, and gestodene are active in their original forms.

In general, the greater a progestin's posthepatic bioavailability, the lower the dosage necessary to inhibit ovulation. Prodrugs that must be metabolized into active form also must be given in higher dosages to compensate for inter- and intraindividual variability.

The progestin dose necessary to inhibit ovulation in combination with 30 to 35 µg EE varies with bioavailability and half-life. Among the gonanes, necessary daily doses range from 30 µg for gestodene to 60 µg for levonorgestrel and desogestrel to 200 µg for norgestimate. The estrane norethindrone requires 400 µg per day.[6]

OC formulations often contain a progestin dose greater than the minimum needed for ovulation inhibition—covering the "margin of error" that results from inter- and intraindividual variability. For example, a combined OC that contains 100 µg levonorgestrel (rather than the 60 µg required for ovulation inhibition) provides a 67% "cushion" to cover the margin of error. Similarly, a combination OC containing 250 µg norgestimate has 25% more progestin than is necessary for ovulation inhibition.

Serum Half-Life

Half-life refers to the time necessary for a drug's blood level to fall to 50% of its maximum. In short, the greater the serum half-life of an OC progestin, the longer the drug lingers in the patient's system. This is desirable from the standpoint of consistent cycle control as well as providing a margin of safety in the event of missed pills.

As with bioavailability, serum half-life of OC progestins has inter- and intraindividual variability. As a consequence of these variations in serum half-life, levonorgestrel and other gonane progestins generally produce better cycle control and less breakthrough bleeding than norethindrone or norethindrone acetate.[1,8,9]

Relative Binding Affinity

A third area in which OC progestins vary widely is their relative binding affinity for the progesterone receptor. The greater the affinity, the smaller the amount of drug necessary for ovulation inhibition.

RBA is usually described as a percentage in relation to a standard reference compound. The most commonly used reference is R5020, a highly potent, synthetic ligand for progesterone receptor analysis.[10] RBA studies have included humans and laboratory animals, such as rabbits.

Many researchers caution against extrapolating the results of animal studies to humans, given the important metabolic differences between species.[1] Differences in OC progestins based on studies in experimental animals cannot be directly extrapolated to human effects; whenever possible, clinical decisions should be based on human data.

A wide variation exists between human and animal data with regard to progestin RBA. Compared with the standard compound R5020 (100%), the relative binding affinity of 3-keto-desogestrel (desogestrel) in the rabbit is 849%; however, its affinity for the human uterine progesterone receptor is considerably lower— 180%. The norgestimate metabolite levonorgestrel-17-acetate also

Figure 7

OC Progestin Pharmacology: Clinical Implications

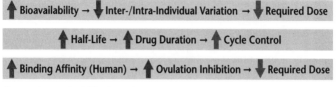

Source: Perone N, 1994 (see reference 1).

has a relatively high affinity in the rabbit, 531%, while its affinity for the human receptor is only one-fifth that amount (110%).[10,11]

Among OC progestins, levonorgestrel has the highest RBA for the human uterine progesterone receptor, 250%. It is followed by the active metabolite of desogestrel, 3-keto-desogestrel (180%).[10] The clinical implications of progestin pharmacology are summarized in Figure 7.

Take Home Messages

■ *Higher bioavailability can result in lower required dosages and less inter- and intraindividual variation*

■ *Long serum half-life is associated with more consistent cycle control and greater contraceptive protection in the event of missed pills*

■ *Greater relative binding affinity means that a smaller dose is needed for a clinical effect*

References

1. Perone N. The progestins. In: Goldzieher JW, Fotherby K, eds. *Pharmacology of the Contraceptive Steroids.* New York: Raven Press; 1994:5-19.

2. Back DJ, Breckenridge AM, Crawford FE, et al. Kinetics of norethindrone in women. II. Single-dose kinetics. *Clin Pharmacol Ther* 1978;24:448-453.

3. Back DJ, Bates M, Breckenridge AM, et al. The pharmacokinetics of levonorgestrel and ethynylestradiol in women—studies with Ovran and Ovranette. *Contraception* 1981;23:229-239.

4. Orme M, Back DJ, Ward S, et al. The pharmacokinetics of ethinyl estradiol in the presence and absence of gestodene and desogestrel. *Contraception* 1991;43:305-316.

5. Stanczyk FZ, Roy S. Metabolism of levonorgestrel, norethindrone, and structurally related contraceptive steroids. *Contraception* 1990;42:67-96.

6. Teichmann AT. Empfangnisverhutung: eine vergleichende Ubersicht aller Methoden, Risiken und Indikationen. Stuttgart, Germany: Georg Thieme Verlag; 1996.

7. Fotherby K, Caldwell ADS. New progestins in oral contraception. *Contraception* 1994;49:1-31.

8. Edgren RA, Nelson JH, Gordon RT, et al. Bleeding patterns with low-dose monophasic oral contraceptives. *Contraception* 1989;40:285-297.

9. Ramos R, Apelo R, Osteria T, et al. A comparative analysis of three different dose combinations of oral contraceptives. *Contraception* 1989;39:165-177.

10. Juchem M, Pollow K, Elger W, et al. Receptor binding of norgestimate— a new orally active synthetic progestational compound. *Contraception* 1993;47:283-294.

11. Phillips A, Demarest K, Hahn DW, et al. Progestational and androgenic receptor binding affinities and in vivo activities of norgestimate and other progestins. *Contraception* 1990;41:399-410.

iii. Androgenicity/Selectivity

Are certain progestins more "androgenic" than others? If so, does this property have clinical relevance, especially when the progestin is combined with estrogen in small, antiovulatory doses? Evidence suggests the answer is no. Neither data nor biologic plausibility support the notion of differing overall OC androgenicity.

Proponents of the notion of differing OC androgenicity often focus on select surrogate markers, an approach which fails to consider the complex system of regulators that ultimately determines androgenic effects.

So-called androgenic effects of progestins probably are more accurately defined as "antiestrogenic." The progestin and estrogen components of combination OCs have differing, sometimes competing, effects on androgen production and free testosterone levels. Progestins tend to counter the estrogenic effects of ethinyl estradiol. The result, however, is a net decrease in endogenous androgens (Figure 8).

Combination OCs prevent ovulation by suppressing follicle-stimulating hormone and luteinizing hormone—their primary contraceptive effect. The suppression of luteinizing hormone by OC progestins results in decreased androgen synthesis by theca cells in the ovary, causing an overall decrease in ovarian androgen (testosterone) production.

Figure 8

Metabolic Effects of Combination Oral Contraceptives: Clinical Implications for Androgen Production and Acne

OC Effect		Clinical Implication
⬇	Luteinizing hormone	Decreased androgen synthesis by theca cells in ovary; net decrease in ovarian androgen production
⬆	Sex hormone-binding globulin	Increased binding of testosterone; lower bioavailability of circulating androgens
⬇	5α-reductase activity	Decreased conversion of testosterone to dihydrotestosterone, the active androgen in hair follicles and skin

OCs also increase sex hormone-binding globulin (SHBG) levels, resulting in increased binding of testosterone. The estrogen component of OCs increases plasma levels of SHBG, while the progestin component has the opposite effect. The overall balance promotes increased liver production of SHBG. In turn, increased SHBG lowers the bioavailability of circulating androgens.

Proponents of the notion of varying androgenicity among OC formulations often point to SHBG levels as support for the concept; however, the steroid-binding system is complex.[1,2] SHBG alone is an insufficient marker for an OC's effect on androgen production. The level of free testosterone is also important in assessing the total level of bioavailable testosterone.[2]

Progestins differ with regard to their ability to inhibit ovarian testosterone production or increase SHBG levels. In general, progestins that are more effective at one function tend to be less effective at the other and vice versa. However, the net effect is similar: combination OCs decrease free testosterone levels by about 40% to 50% in the average woman.[3-5]

In a review of more than 40 studies of the effects of OCs on serum proteins and adrenal steroids, researchers found that nearly all studies reported a drop in free testosterone levels.[3] This decrease took place regardless of whether the pills contained levonorgestrel, norethindrone, gestodene, desogestrel, or norgestimate.

van der Vange et al compared the effects of seven low-dose OC formulations on SHBG, corticosteroid-binding globulin, total testosterone, and free testosterone.[4] Preparations studied included monophasic norethisterone (norethindrone), monophasic levonorgestrel, triphasic levonorgestrel, monophasic desogestrel, biphasic desogestrel, triphasic gestodene, and cyproterone acetate (not available in the US). Although the different formulations raised SHBG levels to varying degrees, they reduced free testosterone by about the same amount.

A recent study by Thorneycroft et al comparing the androgen profiles of two 20 μg EE OCs illustrates this point, as well.[6] Fifty-eight women of reproductive age were randomized to receive either 20 μg EE/100 μg levonorgestrel or 20 μg EE/1 mg norethindrone. Levels of SHBG, total testosterone, and bioavailable testosterone were measured at baseline and at the end of cycle 3. SHBG significantly increased in both groups, although the change was significantly greater in the norethindrone group. On the other hand, only the levonorgestrel group had a significant reduction in total testosterone. Despite this disparity, bioavailable free testosterone and acne (total lesion count) were similarly and significantly reduced in both groups.

In addition, OCs may help decrease conversion of free testosterone to dihydrotestosterone by inhibiting the enzyme 5α-reductase in the hair follicles and skin. Research has indicated that 19-nor-progestins inhibit 5α-reductase activity[7]; OCs containing these progestins may help prevent a key process responsible for androgenic conditions, such as acne and hirsutism.

Testosterone, itself, does nothing to affect acne and hirsutism. Testosterone has to be converted, in the hair follicle and the skin, by 5α-reductase to dihydrotestosterone. At the cellular level, dihydrotestosterone is the active androgen that can increase acne or cause hirsutism. Progestins in oral contraceptives actually inhibit 5α-reductase, an important effect in helping or preventing acne and hirsutism.

Animal Assays and Dose Separation

Misperceptions linger over androgenicity because confusion exists concerning the clinical relevance of preclinical animal assays. Determining the androgenic properties of a progestin traditionally involves an assay that uses immature, castrated male rats. After administering the progestin at various doses, researchers measure the weight increase of the ventral prostate and seminal vesicle. Measurements are compared to the growth induced by testosterone, the "standard" androgen. Increased weight indicates androgenic activity.[8]

Data suggest the amount of progestin required to induce an androgenic activity far exceeds that used in modern OCs. For example, in a dose-separation analysis of levonorgestrel, the dose required to cause an androgenic effect was seven to 200 times greater than the amount needed to suppress ovulation.[9] The dose separation is the difference between the amount needed to achieve the desired effect (ovulation inhibition) and the amount needed to express other properties that may be undesirable.

In clinical terms, the quantity of a progestin (combined with the augmenting effect of the estrogen) needed to inhibit ovulation is so small that androgenic action is simply not expressed. The combination of suppression of the ovaries and the adrenals, and the inhibition of 5α-reductase in the skin and hair follicles, makes such an impact on the endogenous androgen environment that any androgenic action the progestin would have on its own is negligible compared with the overall effect on the body.

Selectivity

Another concept cited in support of suggested differences in OC androgenicity is progestin "selectivity." This theory states that particular progestins may have a greater binding affinity for the uterine progesterone receptor as opposed to others, such as androgen receptors. Proponents argue that the more "selective" a compound is for binding to the desired progesterone receptor, the less binding will occur for undesired receptors, thereby reducing side effects.

What little data exist are, again, from studies using rat prostate.[10] Relative binding affinities in animals and humans have been shown to differ substantially, casting doubt on the clinical relevance of the findings.[8] An extensive review article of new progestins concluded that selectivity is an unproven concept of doubtful relevance because knowledge of how the free steroid interacts with the tissue receptors is limited.[3]

Implications for Acne and Hirsutism

Oral contraceptives improve acne. While clinicians have recognized this benefit for decades, solid evidence from well-done randomized controlled trials only recently became available.[11,12] These studies compared a norgestimate-containing triphasic pill with a placebo as adjunctive therapy for acne and found significant benefit. To date, no randomized trials have compared different OCs in this regard. Other studies, although less rigorous, have found benefit with other types of pills, as would be expected from their hormonal effects. OCs increase SHGB, which, in turn, lowers free testosterone. Given this effect of all combined OCs on androgens, the hypothesis that various pills differ importantly in "androgenicity" lacks a scientific basis. (For further discussion of OCs as treatment for acne, see the section on use of OCs to treat medical disorders.)

Take Home Messages

- *Combination OCs suppress ovarian, adrenal, and peripheral androgen metabolism, resulting in a net reduction in free testosterone*

- *OCs inhibit 5α-reductase in the skin, resulting in lower levels of the active androgen dihydrotestosterone*

- *Data show that many OCs containing various progestins help reduce androgen-related conditions, such as acne and hirsutism*

- *Evidence does not support any distinction among combination OC formulations with regard to androgen-related conditions*

References

1. Rosner W. Plasma steroid-binding proteins. *Endocrinol Metab Clin North Am* 1991;20:697-720.

2. Rosner W, Hryb DJ, Khan MS, et al. Sex hormone-binding globulin: anatomy and physiology of a new regulatory system. *J Steroid Biochem Mol Biol* 1991;40:813-820.

3. Fotherby K, Caldwell ADS. New progestins in oral contraception. *Contraception* 1994;49:1-32.

4. van der Vange N, Blankenstein MA, Kloosterboer HJ, et al. Effects of seven low-dose oral contraceptives on sex hormone binding globulin, corticosteroid binding globulin, total and free testosterone. *Contraception* 1990;41: 345-352.

5. Thorneycroft IH. Update on androgenicity. *Am J Obstet Gynecol* 1999;180: S288-S294.

6. Thorneycroft IH, Stanczyk FZ, Bradshaw KD, et al. Effect of low-dose oral contraceptives on androgenic markers and acne. *Contraception* 1999;60: 255-262.

7. Cassidenti DL, Paulson RJ, Serafini P, et al. Effects of sex steroids on skin 5α-reductase activity in vitro. *Obstet Gynecol* 1991;78:103-107.

8. Goldzieher JW. *Hormonal Contraception: Pills, Injections & Implants.* 4th ed. Ontario: EMIS-CANADA; 1998.

9. Upton GV, Corbin A. The relevance of the pharmacologic properties of a progestational agent to its clinical effects as a combination oral contraceptive. *Yale J Biol Med* 1989;62:445-457.

10. Phillips A, Demarest K, Hahn DW, et al. Progestational and androgenic receptor binding affinities and in vivo activities of norgestimate and other progestins. *Contraception* 1990;41:399-410.

11. Redmond GP, Olson WH, Lippman JS, et al. Norgestimate and ethinyl estradiol in the treatment of acne vulgaris: a randomized, placebo-controlled trial. *Obstet Gynecol* 1997;89:615-622.

12. Lucky AW, Henderson TA, Olson WH, et al. Effectiveness of norgestimate and ethinyl estradiol in treating moderate acne vulgaris. *J Am Acad Dermatol* 1997;37:746-754.

1.6: Medical Eligibility Criteria

In 1996, the World Health Organization (WHO) released revised medical eligibility criteria guidelines to assist family planning agencies and clinicians in prescribing contraceptive methods.[1] The primary goal was to improve access to contraception without causing undue risk to patients. One concern was that women were inappropriately being denied oral contraceptives. Systematic evaluation of the scientific evidence has resulted in a more thorough understanding of low-dose OC safety. Many of the "standard" prescribing contraindications listed in the package labeling are outdated and based on early, often flawed, studies of high-dose OCs.

Medical problems do not necessarily preclude use of combination OCs. In situations in which women have preexisting medical conditions, the theoretical or known risk of the method must be weighed against the benefit of preventing a potentially high-risk pregnancy. WHO researchers evaluated the benefits and risks of using combination OCs in healthy, nonsmoking women and in women with certain medical conditions or individual characteristics, such as age, parity, and family history. The eligibility criteria were developed by international experts from many organizations after a thorough review of the medical literature. Several tables adapted from the WHO guidelines provide a sampling of the various issues addressed by WHO.

Women may be denied access to effective contraception if policies are based on outdated medical information. According to WHO, "Over the past 30 years, there have been significant advances in the development of new contraceptive technologies, including transitions from high-dose to low-dose combined oral contraceptives. ...Current policies and health care practices in some countries are based on scientific studies of contraceptive products that are no longer in wide use, on long-standing theoretical concerns that have never been substantiated, or on the personal preference or bias of service providers. These outdated policies or practices many times result in limitations to both the quality of, and the access to, family planning services."

Reexamining Contraindications

Some agencies and health care providers create barriers to access by having unreasonable checklists of contraindications before providing contraceptives. WHO cautions that "The contraindications for many contraceptives tend to become very rigid, resulting in denial of contraceptive access to many women. Relative contraindications tend to become absolute." For example, many conditions, such as thyroid disease, trophoblastic disease, sickle cell anemia, and varicose veins, are incorrectly considered contraindications to the use of combination OCs.

Similarly, unexplained vaginal bleeding has become an "abused" contraindication. In countries where easy access to pregnancy testing or routine examination is unavailable, unexplained vaginal bleeding indicates the need for an assessment for pregnancy or malignancy. Thus, irregular vaginal bleeding, in and of itself, is not truly a contraindication to OC use. The presence of headaches is also overused as a contraindication. The WHO experts defined more specifically the conditions in which severe headaches should be considered a contraindication for combination OC use: namely, if accompanied by focal neurological symptoms. (For further discussion, see the section on OCs and headache/migraine.)

WHO guidelines help to simplify screening measures for contraceptive use. For example, routine lipid screening, urinalysis, and glucose tests are not necessary for the provision of OCs. On the other hand, a careful history and blood pressure measurement are highly recommended.

Balancing Risks and Benefits

The new WHO categorization process guides clinicians in the choice of contraceptive by balancing the risks and benefits of the method under certain conditions (Table 6). For example, if the presence of a particular condition creates no obstacle to use, the condition receives a Category 1 rating. If the benefits of a method generally outweigh the risks, the condition receives a Category 2 rating. Category 3 applies to conditions carrying risks that generally outweigh benefits, whereas Category 4 applies to conditions carrying unacceptable health risks.

One advantage of the WHO system is that it can be applied when clinical expertise is limited. For example, Categories 1 and 2 can be applied by personnel without substantial medical knowledge. On the other hand, if the woman's condition falls into Category 3, it may be best not to use that method unless a clinician who can exercise greater judgment is available.

The numerical category determination for each condition reflects WHO's evaluation of the quality and strength of the evidence. The quality of information depends upon the type of study, criteria for establishing causality, and other criteria used to evaluate case-control and cohort studies. Evidence from properly designed, randomized controlled trials receive the most weight, while evidence obtained from nonrandomized controlled trials and case-control studies receive less weight. Factors considered in

Table 6

WHO Rating Criteria

Classification	Eligibility Category	Use When Clinical Judgment Available	Use When Limited Clinical Judgment Available
1	A condition for which there is no restriction for the use of the contraceptive method.	Use method in any circumstance.	Yes
2	A condition in which the advantages of using the method generally outweigh the theoretical or proven risks.	Generally use the method.	Yes
3	A condition in which the theoretical or proven risks usually outweigh the advantages of using the method.	Use of method not usually recommended unless other, more appropriate, methods are not available or not acceptable.	No
4	A condition which represents unacceptable health risk if the contraceptive method is used.	Method not to be used.	No

Source: World Health Organization, 1996 (see reference 1).

establishing causality include the strength of the association, biological plausibility, and dose-response relationship, among others.

The WHO guidelines clarify prescribing guidelines for women with various medical conditions. For example, WHO guidelines suggest that the benefits of combination OCs generally outweigh the risks for diabetic women, whether insulin dependent or not, as long as they are free of serious cardiovascular complications. The investigators suggest caution or no use (Category 3 or 4) for diabetic women with vascular disease or diabetes of greater than 20 years' duration. Table 7 lists Category 3 conditions (risks may outweigh the benefits of OC use). Table 8 lists those conditions WHO rates as Category 4 (method presents unacceptable health risks).

WHO guidelines suggest a Category 1 and 2 rating for varicose veins and superficial venous thrombosis, respectively. Only a history of deep venous thrombosis precludes combination OC use.

WHO researchers make a clear distinction between irregular vaginal bleeding and *unexplained* vaginal bleeding. Irregular bleeding patterns are quite common among healthy women. Irregular menstrual periods, with or without heavy or prolonged bleeding, fall into Category 1. On the other hand, unexplained vaginal bleeding may require evaluation for an underlying pathological condition. During the evaluation, OCs can be continued in a woman already taking them (Category 2). Women who are just beginning OCs probably should wait for the results of the evaluation before starting the method (Category 3).

Other conditions for which OCs may be used with no restrictions include the presence of sexually transmitted diseases (including HIV infection or AIDS), current or past pelvic inflammatory disease, family history of breast cancer, recent abortion, history of ectopic pregnancy, trophoblastic disease, thalassemia, schistosomiasis, and thyroid disease.

Take Home Messages

- *WHO guidelines can help clinicians balance the risks and benefits of using OCs for women with certain medical conditions*
- *WHO prescribing guidelines are based on an evaluation of the quality and strength of the evidence*

Table 7

WHO Guidelines: Conditions Under Which Combined OC Use Is Generally Not Recommended

*Category 3**

- *Hypertension*

  - *History of hypertension in which BP** cannot be monitored (excluding hypertension in pregnancy)*

  - *BP 160-179/100-109 mmHg – initiate use of OCs with caution and only if regular monitoring available and no additional risk factors*

  - *BP 140-159/90-99 mmHg is a Category 2/3, depending upon risk factors and availability of monitoring‡*

- *Diabetes with retinopathy/nephropathy/neuropathy or with other vascular disease or disease duration >20 years (Category 3/4, depending upon severity)*

- *Smoking (up to 20 cigarettes/day) and age ≥35 years*

- *Mild cirrhosis*

- *Postpartum <21 days*

- *Breastfeeding, 6 weeks to 6 months (primarily breastfeeding)§*

- *Past breast cancer with no evidence of disease for 5 years†*

- *Unexplained suspicious vaginal bleeding (before evaluation)*

- *Long-term use of enzyme-inducing antibiotics or anticonvulsants*

- *History of OC-related cholestasis*

- *Symptomatic biliary tract disease (current or treated medically)*

- *Known genetic hyperlipidemias (Category 2/3, depending upon type and severity)*

* Category 3: use of method not usually recommended unless other, more appropriate methods are not available or not acceptable. (For further discussion, see the section on use of OCs for women with medical disorders.)

** Blood pressure

‡ Borderline and mild high blood pressure values are lower among teens.

§ WHO recommendations regarding low-dose combined OCs and breastfeeding are conservative and controversial. (For further discussion, see the section on breastfeeding.)

† WHO recommendations are based on theoretical concerns, but no data are available.

Source: World Health Organization, 1996 (see reference 1).

Table 8

WHO Guidelines: Conditions Under Which Combined OCs Should Not Be Used

*Category 4**

- *Pregnancy*
- *History of or current ischemic heart disease*
- *History of stroke*
- *History of or current deep venous thrombosis or pulmonary embolism*
- *Vascular disease*
- *Complicated valvular heart disease (pulmonary hypertension, atrial fibrillation, history of subacute bacterial endocarditis)*
- *Hypertension: BP** of ≥180/110 mmHg*
  BP of 160-179/100-109 mmHg warrants OC discontinuation in a current user
- *Smoking >20 cigarettes/day and age ≥35 years*
- *Migraine headache with focal neurologic symptoms*
- *Major surgery with prolonged immobilization*
- *Current breast cancer*
- *Active viral hepatitis[†]*
- *Severe (decompensated) cirrhosis*
- *Benign or malignant liver tumors*
- *Breastfeeding, <6 weeks postpartum*

* Category 4: method not to be used.

** Blood pressure

[†] Some data published since WHO's recommendations indicate that treatment with 20 µg ethinyl estradiol significantly improved serum enzyme levels in six women with chronic inflammatory hepatitis.[2]

Source: World Health Organization, 1996 (see reference 1).

Table 9

WHO Guidelines: Conditions Under Which Combined OCs May Be Used Without Restriction

Condition	Category	Rationale/Comments
POSTABORTION		
a) First trimester	1	OCs may be started immediately postabortion.
b) Second trimester	1	
c) Post-septic abortion	1	
SUPERFICIAL VENOUS THROMBOSIS		
a) Varicose veins	1	
b) Superficial thrombophlebitis	2	
THALASSEMIAS	2	OCs may induce the development of specific metabolic disorders.
VAGINAL BLEEDING PATTERNS		
a) Irregular pattern *without* heavy bleeding	1	Changes in menstrual bleeding patterns are common among healthy women. OCs may decrease menstrual blood loss.
b) Irregular patterns *with* heavy or prolonged bleeding (includes regular patterns)	1	

UNEXPLAINED VAGINAL BLEEDING (suspicious for serious condition)			
	Initiation	Continuation	
Before evaluation	3	2	If pregnancy or an underlying pathological condition (such as pelvic malignancy) is suspected, it must be evaluated and the category adjusted after evaluation.

UTERINE FIBROIDS	1	OCs do not cause growth of uterine fibroids.

WHO Guidelines: Conditions Under Which Combined OCs May Be Used Without Restriction
continued

Condition	Category	Rationale/Comments
PAST ECTOPIC PREGNANCY	1	The risk of future ectopic pregnancy is increased among women who have had an ectopic pregnancy. OCs provide protection against ectopic pregnancy.
OBESITY	1	Obesity is not relevant for this contraceptive method.
THYROID a) Simple goiter	1	The condition is not relevant for eligibility for this contraceptive method.
b) Hyperthyroid	1	
c) Hypothyroid	1	
TROPHOBLASTIC DISEASE a) Benign gestational trophoblastic disease	1	There is no concern about progression of the disease with OC use. The woman needs a highly effective contraceptive method.
b) Malignant gestational trophoblastic disease	1	
PARITY a) Nulliparous	1	There is no need for restriction of OC use for nulliparous or parous women.
b) Parous	1	
SEVERE DYSMENORRHEA	1	OC use may decrease or alleviate symptoms of dysmenorrhea.

WHO Guidelines: Conditions Under Which Combined OCs May Be Used Without Restriction
continued

Condition	Category	Rationale/Comments
TUBERCULOSIS		
a) Nonpelvic	1	Prognosis of tuberculosis is not affected by the use of OCs (see the section on drug interactions).
b) Known pelvic	1	
ENDOMETRIOSIS	1	OCs do not worsen endometriosis. OCs may alleviate the symptoms of endometriosis.
BENIGN OVARIAN TUMORS (including cysts)	1	Benign ovarian tumors are not affected by OC use.
PRIOR PELVIC SURGERY	1	Prior pelvic surgery has no effect on OC use.
BREAST DISEASE		
a) Undiagnosed mass	2	The vast majority of breast masses in women of reproductive age are benign. Evaluation should be pursued as early as possible.
b) Benign breast disease	1	The condition is not relevant for eligibility for this contraceptive method.
c) Family history of cancer	1	Not related to OC use for women with benign breast disease or family history of breast disease.
d) Cancer *current*	4	Breast cancer is a hormonally sensitive tumor. The risk for progress of the condition may be increased among women taking hormones.
past and no evidence of current disease for 5 years	3	

WHO Guidelines: Conditions Under Which Combined OCs May Be Used Without Restriction
continued

Condition	Category	Rationale/Comments
HISTORY OF PREECLAMPSIA	1	Absence of underlying vascular disease suggests no need for restriction of OC use.
POSTPARTUM (in nonbreastfeeding women)		
a) <21 days	3	Blood coagulation and fibrinolysis are essentially normalized by 3 weeks postpartum.
b) ≥21 days	1	
SURGERY		
a) Major surgery		
with prolonged immobilization	4	
without prolonged immobilization	2	
b) Minor surgery without immobilization	1	
VIRAL HEPATITIS		
a) Active	4	Because OCs are metabolized by the liver, their use may adversely affect women whose liver function is already compromised.
b) Carrier	1	
KNOWN HYPERLIPIDEMIAS	2/3	Some types of hyperlipidemias are risk factors for vascular disease. However, the category should be assessed according to the type and its severity. Routine screening is not appropriate because of the rarity of the conditions and the high cost of screening.

Source: World Health Organization, 1996 (see reference 1).

To obtain the document *Improving Access to Quality Care in Family Planning. Medical Eligibility Criteria for Contraceptive Use,* contact (in New York):

WHO Publications Center

Phone number: 518-436-9686, Extension 118

The publication is available for $18.00 plus $5.00 shipping and handling. Prepayment is required.

References

1.   Family and Reproductive Health Programme. *Improving Access to Quality Care in Family Planning. Medical Eligibility Criteria for Contraceptive Use.* Geneva: World Health Organization; 1996:1-30.

2.   Guattery JM, Faloon WW, Beiry DL. Effect of ethinyl estradiol on chronic active hepatitis. *Ann Intern Med* 1997;126:88. Letter.

1.7: Current Formulations

Several classifications of oral contraceptives exist. The "strength" of combined OCs reflects the estrogen dose, with 50 μg of ethinyl estradiol defining "high dose" and <50 μg defining "low dose." The classification by regimen indicates whether the estrogen and progestin vary during the cycle; for example, mono-, bi-, and triphasic. Another classification of OCs includes brand-name products vs generic formulations.

Today's "High-" and "Low-Dose" OCs

- High-dose — contain 50 μg ethinyl estradiol.
- Low-dose — contain 20, 30, or 35 μg ethinyl estradiol or 50 μg mestranol.

Early OCs contained high doses of both hormones by contemporary standards. For example, early formulations contained the equivalent of about 80 to 100 μg ethinyl estradiol. Doses of estrogen have dropped to one-third or one-quarter of their original dose. Early formulations also contained high doses of progestin — up to 10 mg of norethindrone. That dose has now been reduced to one-tenth or less of the original (500 μg to 1 mg). About 99% of all OC prescriptions today are written for formulations containing ≤35 μg of estrogen.

Phasing

Varying the amount of estrogen or progestin in the OC has become common. Today's OCs are often classified by whether the doses of hormone are constant or variable.

- Monophasic — monophasic OCs have constant doses of both estrogen and progestin.
- Multiphasic — multiphasic OCs contain varying doses of progestin, estrogen, or both. Both triphasic and biphasic OCs are available, although biphasic formulations are rarely used in the US.
  - Triphasic — triphasic OCs vary the dose of progestin or estrogen in three phases.

 – Biphasic — biphasic OCs contain 10 days of one dose of progestin and then 11 days of another dose, with the estrogen
 remaining constant.

In 1998, a low-dose OC came on the market that alters the traditional 7-day pill-free interval (20 µg EE plus 0.15 mg deso-gestrel). This 20 µg OC shortens the hormone-free interval to only 2 days and then resumes the rest of the traditional pill-free week with 10 µg estrogen. Table 10 identifies OCs available in the United States. (See Appendix B for a list of low-dose OCs available in Canada.)

Although various claims have been made concerning the benefits of phasing either the estrogen or progestin, the evidence is unclear. A total reduction in steroid dose has been achieved compared with some monophasic products, although not all. Triphasics have different colored pills, which may be confusing to some women. A Cochrane Collaboration review of all the random-ized controlled trials of multi- vs monophasic OCs is under way now and may clarify these issues. Cochrane reviews are evidence-based, systematic reviews of randomized controlled trials of medical practices.

Generic OCs

The Food and Drug Administration (FDA) has approved several generic OCs. FDA approval is based on small studies (20 to 30 subjects) of serum bioequivalence. Generic OCs must have 80% to 125% bioequivalence of branded products.[1] Whether failure rates might be higher with generic OCs is unknown. No data are available regarding efficacy in a large population of users, unlike brand-name OCs.

Reference
1.   Williams RL. Therapeutic equivalence of generic drugs. Response to National
      Association of Boards of Pharmacy. US FDA Center for Drug Evaluation and
      Research; 1998. Available at: http://www.fda.gov/cder/news/ntiletter.htm.
      Accessed December 9, 1999.

Table 10 provides, in alphabetical order, the name, steroid content, and manufacturer of OCs currently on the US market. The table identifies OCs by estrogen dose. The table also further subdivides OCs into monophasic, multiphasic, and progestin-only preparations and identifies the OC by the type of progestin —either gonane or estrane.

Table 10

Oral Contraceptives Available in the United States

Product Name*	Manufacturer	Estrogen	μg	Progestin	mg
Monophasic preparations					
20 μg estrogen					
Gonane progestin					
Alesse	Wyeth-Ayerst	EE	20	Levonorgestrel	0.10
Levlite	Berlex	EE	20	Levonorgestrel	0.10
Estrane progestin					
Loestrin 1/20	Parke-Davis	EE	20	Norethindrone acetate	1.00
Loestrin Fe 1/20	Parke-Davis	EE	20	Norethindrone acetate	1.00
30-35 μg estrogen					
Gonane progestin					
Desogen	Organon	EE	30	Desogestrel	0.15
Levlen	Berlex	EE	30	Levonorgestrel	0.15
Levora	Watson	EE	30	Levonorgestrel	0.15
Lo/Ovral	Wyeth-Ayerst	EE	30	Norgestrel	0.30

EE = ethinyl estradiol Mes = mestranol
* Product names are for identification purposes only and do not imply endorsement.
** ( ) = number of days each dosage is taken.

41

Oral Contraceptives Available in the United States *continued*

Product Name*	Manufacturer	Estrogen	µg	Progestin	mg
Low-Ogestrel	SCS Pharmaceuticals	EE	30	Norgestrel	0.30
Nordette	Wyeth-Ayerst	EE	30	Levonorgestrel	0.15
Ortho-Cept	Ortho-McNeil	EE	30	Desogestrel	0.15
Estrane progestin					
Brevicon	Searle	EE	35	Norethindrone	0.50
Demulen 1/35	Searle	EE	35	Ethynodiol diacetate	1.00
Loestrin 1.5/30	Parke-Davis	EE	30	Norethindrone acetate	1.50
Loestrin Fe 1.5/30	Parke-Davis	EE	30	Norethindrone acetate	1.50
Modicon	Ortho-McNeil	EE	35	Norethindrone	0.50
Necon 0.5/35	Watson	EE	35	Norethindrone	0.50
Necon 1/35	Watson	EE	35	Norethindrone	1.00
Nelova 0.5/35E	Warner Chilcott	EE	35	Norethindrone	0.50
Nelova 1/35E	Warner Chilcott	EE	35	Norethindrone	1.00
Norinyl 1 + 35	Searle	EE	35	Norethindrone	1.00
Ortho-Cyclen	Ortho-McNeil	EE	35	Norgestimate	0.25
Ortho-Novum 1/35	Ortho-McNeil	EE	35	Norethindrone	1.00
Ovcon-35	Bristol-Myers Squibb	EE	35	Norethindrone	0.40
Zovia 1/35E	Watson	EE	35	Ethynodiol diacetate	1.00

Oral Contraceptives Available in the United States *continued*

Product Name*	Manufacturer	Estrogen	μg	Progestin	mg
50 μg estrogen					
Gonane progestin					
Ovral	Wyeth-Ayerst	EE	50	Norgestrel	0.50
Estrane progestin					
Demulen 1/50	Searle	EE	50	Ethynodiol diacetate	1.00
Necon 1/50***	Watson	Mes	50	Norethindrone	1.00
Nelova 1/50M***	Warner Chilcott	Mes	50	Norethindrone	1.00
Norinyl 1 + 50***	Searle	Mes	50	Norethindrone	1.00
Ortho-Novum 1/50***	Ortho-McNeil	Mes	50	Norethindrone	1.00
Ovcon 50	Bristol-Myers Squibb	EE	50	Norethindrone	1.00
Zovia 1/50E	Watson	EE	50	Ethynodiol diacetate	1.00
Multiphasic preparations					
20 μg estrogen					
Gonane progestin					
Mircette	Organon	EE	20 (21)** 0 (2) 10 (5)	Desogestrel	0.15

EE = ethinyl estradiol Mes = mestranol

  * Product names are for identification purposes only and do not imply endorsement.

 ** ( ) = number of days each dosage is taken.

*** A 50 μg OC containing mestranol is bioequivalent to a 35 μg EE OC because about 30% of mestranol is lost in the conversion to ethinyl estradiol.

Oral Contraceptives Available in the United States *continued*

Product Name*	Manufacturer	Estrogen	μg	Progestin	mg
30-35 μg estrogen					
Gonane progestin					
Ortho Tri-Cyclen	Ortho-McNeil	EE	35 (21)**	Norgestimate	0.18 (7)
				Norgestimate	0.215 (7)
				Norgestimate	0.25 (7)
Tri-Levlen	Berlex	EE	30 (6)	Levonorgestrel	0.05 (6)
		EE	40 (5)	Levonorgestrel	0.075 (5)
		EE	30 (10)	Levonorgestrel	0.125 (10)
Triphasil	Wyeth-Ayerst	EE	30 (6)	Levonorgestrel	0.05 (6)
		EE	40 (5)	Levonorgestrel	0.075 (5)
		EE	30 (10)	Levonorgestrel	0.125 (10)
Trivora	Watson	EE	30 (6)	Levonorgestrel	0.05 (6)
		EE	40 (5)	Levonorgestrel	0.075 (5)
		EE	30 (10)	Levonorgestrel	0.125 (10)
Estrane progestin					
Estrostep	Parke-Davis	EE	20 (5)	Norethindrone acetate	1.00
		EE	30 (7)		
		EE	35 (9)		
Estrostep Fe	Parke-Davis	EE	20 (5)	Norethindrone acetate	1.00
		EE	30 (7)		
		EE	35 (9)		

EE = ethinyl estradiol Mes = mestranol
* Product names are for identification purposes only and do not imply endorsement.
** ( ) = number of days each dosage is taken.

Oral Contraceptives Available in the United States *continued*

Product Name*	Manufacturer	Estrogen	μg	Progestin	mg
Jenest	Organon	EE	35 (21)**	Norethindrone	0.50 (7)
					1.00 (14)
Necon 10/11	Watson	EE	35 (21)	Norethindrone	0.50 (10)
					1.00 (11)
Nelova 10/11	Warner Chilcott	EE	35 (21)	Norethindrone	0.50 (10)
					1.00 (11)
Ortho-Novum 10/11	Ortho-McNeil	EE	35 (21)	Norethindrone	0.50 (10)
					1.00 (11)
Ortho-Novum 7/7/7	Ortho-McNeil	EE	35 (21)	Norethindrone	0.50 (7)
					0.75 (7)
					1.00 (7)
Tri-Norinyl	Searle	EE	35 (21)	Norethindrone	0.50 (7)
					1.00 (9)
					0.50 (5)

Progestin only

Gonane progestin

Ovrette	Wyeth-Ayerst	None		Norgestrel	0.075

Estrane progestin

Micronor	Ortho-McNeil	None		Norethindrone	0.35
Nor-QD	Watson	None		Norethindrone	0.35

EE = ethinyl estradiol   Mes = mestranol
* Product names are for identification purposes only and do not imply endorsement.
** ( ) = number of days each dosage is taken.

1.8: General Principles of Prescribing

US clinicians have about 40 brands of low-dose oral contraceptives from which to choose. Clinicians may be overwhelmed by the number of choices and may wonder if a "scientific" rationale for using one type of pill rather than another exists. A few have attempted such systems.[1,2] Data are sparse, however, to suggest any of these classifications is scientifically justified.

Individual Differences in Steroid Metabolism

An important, but often underrecognized, element of prescribing OCs is the large inter- and intraindividual differences in steroid metabolism among women. Pharmacokinetic investigations have shown large variations, both between women and within the same woman, in how the body metabolizes both estrogen and progestin.[3,4] Therefore, how a particular woman will react to a particular OC formulation is impossible to predict.

Lipids, Potency, and Androgenicity

Over the years, approaches to prescribing have emphasized specific aspects of OC metabolism or side effects. For example, for many years, an OC's effect on lipids was a criterion used to judge the desirability of the particular formulation. A widely held notion suggested that adverse lipid effects induced by OCs could result in an increased risk of cardiovascular disease among women. That theory came into question, however, when data suggested that the estrogen in OCs helps to prevent atherosclerotic plaque formation despite adverse changes in lipids. (For further discussion, see the section on metabolic effects of OCs.) In addition, data suggested that cardiovascular events in OC users were thrombotic, rather than atherogenic, in nature. Thus, the admonition to prescribe one OC over another based on the effect on lipids had little supporting evidence.

Another theory, briefly popular in the early 1980s, suggested that OC formulations had inherently different "potencies." Some speculated that the potency of a given formulation was linked to breast cancer among women using OCs.[5] This hypothesis was rejected by the US Food and Drug Administration in 1985.

In addition, progestins used in OCs have been compared according to their "relative potency." The issue, however, is often misunderstood. When measuring the potency of a progestin, researchers assess the action of the compound on the estrogen-primed endometrium. However, results from these types of assessments should not be used to determine the "relative potencies" of progestins because there is no assurance that the data derived are comparable when the compounds are tested in another organ or tissue.

The latest confusion concerns the labeling of certain OCs as "androgenic."[1,2,6] Describing OCs by the supposed androgenicity of the progestin is misleading for the following reasons:

1. All combination OCs suppress ovarian and adrenal androgen production;

2. The overall effect of all combination OCs is a decreased androgen environment;

3. Animal assays, often used to determine androgenicity, have limited clinical relevance; and,

4. The suppression of 5α-reductase in the skin and hair follicles helps to decrease acne and hirsutism.

(For further discussion, see the section on OC progestins and androgenicity.)

Some prescribing recommendations have provided tables labeling the "relative potency" and estrogenic, progestational, and androgenic properties of various OCs.[1,2] These guidelines are largely based on opinion and animal data that cannot be extrapolated to humans. The assessment of potency of both estrogen and progestin is exceedingly complex because bioassays can be influenced by species, target organ or tissue, temporal variables, route of administration, and enterohepatic circulation.[7] Progestational agents alone have over 25 biologic effects.[7] The reliability, validity, and clinical relevance of potency estimates are highly questionable, as are prescribing guidelines based on these ratings.

Choosing an OC

Selecting an oral contraceptive formulation for a particular woman is largely a matter of availability of formulations, cost considerations, history of past OC use, and clinical experience. The large inter- and intraindividual differences in steroid metabolism preclude predicting clinical performance. The following general guidelines may be helpful.

Past History of OC Use

If the woman has used OCs successfully in the past and was happy with the pill formulation, then that OC may be a good choice for her. The clinician may want to prescribe the same OC.

Side Effects During Past OC Use

If the woman experienced estrogen-related side effects, such as nausea, breast tenderness, or bloating, the clinician may want to use a lower dose of estrogen; for example, choosing a 20 μg rather than a 30 or 35 μg OC. If the woman has a history of breakthrough bleeding, a higher estrogen dose may be used. On the other hand, if the side effects were progestin-related, such as perceived mood changes, the clinician may want to use an OC with a different type of progestin (estrane vs gonane) or less progestin.

Conditions Related to the Menstrual Cycle

Some women may experience premenstrual syndrome, menstrual migraine, or seizures that worsen during menses. Some clinicians keep such women on active, monophasic OCs for 90 days, then allow a withdrawal bleed and repeat.[8]

Drug Interactions

Women who are using enzyme-inducing medications long term, such as rifampin, griseofulvin, or certain anticonvulsants, may metabolize the hormones in OCs more rapidly and, possibly, be subjected to an increased risk of pregnancy or breakthrough bleeding. (For further discussion, see the sections on epilepsy and drug interactions.)

Encouraging 3 Months of OC Use Before Switching

Because nuisance side effects, such as nausea and breakthrough bleeding, commonly disappear within 3 months of beginning OC use, the clinician should make every effort not to switch formulations until after a 3-month trial.

Weighing Risk vs Benefit

In all women, the risks and benefits of OCs need to be carefully weighed against a potential unintended pregnancy. The woman's smoking status, other medical conditions, and willingness to use another method should be taken into consideration. Medical concerns about OC use need to be weighed against the known risks of pregnancy. (For further discussion, see the section on use of OCs in women with medical disorders.)

Take Home Messages

- *How a particular woman will react to a particular OC formulation is impossible to predict*
- *Approaches to prescribing OCs based on lipid effects, "potency," and "androgenicity" are not supported by the evidence*
- *Selecting an OC formulation for a particular woman is largely a matter of availability, cost considerations, history of OC use, and clinical experience*

References

1. Dickey RP. *Managing Contraceptive Pill Patients.* 9th ed. Durant, Oklahoma: EMIS, Inc.; 1998.

2. Mishell DR Jr. Practice guidelines for OC selection: update. *Dialogues in Contraception* 1997;5:7-20.

3. Fotherby K. Pharmacokinetics and metabolism of progestins in humans. In: Goldzieher JW, Fotherby K, eds. *Pharmacology of the Contraceptive Steroids.* New York: Raven Press; 1994:99-126.

4. Goldzieher JW. Pharmacokinetics and metabolism of ethynyl estrogens. In: Goldzieher JW, Fotherby K, eds. *Pharmacology of the Contraceptive Steroids.* New York: Raven Press; 1994:127-141.

5. Pike MC, Henderson BE, Krailo MD, et al. Breast cancer in young women and use of oral contraceptives: possible modifying effect of formulation and age at use. *Lancet* 1983;2:926-930.

6. Darney PD. OC practice guidelines: minimizing side effects. *Int J Fertil Womens Med* 1997;(suppl 1):158-169.

7.   Goldzieher JW. Use and misuse of the term *potency* with respect to oral con-
      traceptives. *J Reprod Med* 1986;31(suppl):533-537.

8.   Sulak PJ, Cressman BE, Waldrop E, et al. Extending the duration of active
      oral contraceptive pills to manage hormone withdrawal symptoms. *Obstet
      Gynecol* 1997;89:179-183.

1.9: Starting OCs

Clinicians generally follow one of two routines for starting OCs: a Sunday start or starting on the first day of the menstrual cycle. Another practice is starting oral contraceptives on the day that the OC is prescribed, regardless of the time in the menstrual cycle. Data regarding the impact of this choice are not available.

Sunday Start

Women beginning OCs with a Sunday start take their first OC pill on the first Sunday after the menstrual cycle begins. If menstruation begins on a Sunday, the woman should take her first OC pill that day. No backup method of contraception is necessary. If her period begins on a day other than Sunday, however, she should use a backup method of contraception until having taken the first week of pills.

One advantage of a Sunday start for large clinics is all patients start on the same day, making more consistent counseling possible. Another advantage is that pill taking corresponds to calendar weeks. One difficulty that may occur with a Sunday start, however, is getting a new prescription of pills filled on a weekend. The concept of starting OCs on a Sunday was originally developed so women would not have their periods on the weekend.

First-Day Start

First-day starters begin taking OCs on the first day of their menstrual cycle, regardless of the day of the week. With the first-day start, women do not need to use a backup method of contraception.

Quick Start

In the quick-start method, women begin the OC regimen on the day they come in for their examination and prescription. One advantage of this regimen is that the patient doesn't have to remember the starting instructions for OCs. On the other hand, a woman who starts OCs midcycle will need to use backup contraception for 1 week. In addition, irregular bleeding may be more likely when starting OCs midcycle, which may hurt compliance. One concern is that the quick start approach may delay the diagnosis of pregnancy; however, women can be reassured that low-dose OCs will not harm a developing embryo.

Family Health International recommends the following for beginning oral contraceptives using the quick-start method.[1]

Combination OCs

- OCs may be started at any time in a woman who is reasonably sure she's not pregnant and who has not recently given birth.
- When combination OCs are begun within the first 7 days of the menstrual cycle, the woman does not need to use a backup method of contraception.
- Women starting combination OCs after day 7 of the menstrual cycle should use a backup method of contraception for the first cycle.

Starting Combination OCs Postpartum or Postabortion

Postpartum

- Breastfeeding — women who are breastfeeding may use combination OCs once lactation is well established.
- Nonbreastfeeding — women who elect not to breastfeed may begin using combination OCs at 3 weeks postpartum.

(For further discussion, refer to the sections on breastfeeding and progestin-only OCs.)

Postabortion

- After abortion, women may begin OCs immediately.

Missed Pills

Instructions for what to do about missed pills vary among organizations and individual clinicians. In the case of one missed pill, the instructions are consistent. The woman should take the forgotten pill as soon as she remembers; the next pill should be taken at the regular time. In the case of missing two pills, the instructions differ, depending upon when in the cycle the pills are missed. If the woman misses three or more pills in a row, the instructions are generally consistent. The woman should keep taking active pills and abstain from sex or use a backup method of contraception for 7 days after missing pills.

In 1991, the FDA's Fertility and Maternal Health Drugs Advisory Committee unanimously agreed to accept revised patient package insert instructions developed by Family Health International.[2] By April 1992, manufacturers had revised labeling. Patient package inserts now include standardized instructions about what to do in case of missed pills (summarized by Goldzieher[3] in Table 11). On the other hand, updated guidelines for missed pills published in 1996 do not distinguish among missing two, three, or more pills, or between a Sunday or first-day start (Table 12).[1]

Because instructions about what to do in case of missed pills can be complex, a further simplified guide for patients may be useful (Table 13). These instructions do not recommend backup contraception among women who miss two active pills. Data indicate that escape ovulation is most likely to occur at the end of an extended (more than 7 days) pill-free interval.[4-10] An extended pill-free interval occurs when one or more pills are missed just prior to or immediately following the 7-day pill-free week. At other times in the cycle, the risk of pregnancy escalates substantially only when three or more pills are missed.

Some data suggest that extending the pill-free week by three or even four missed pills may not result in ovulation.[11,12] A randomized trial monitored ovarian activity in 99 women using low-dose OCs containing either gestodene or desogestrel during two cycles of use (one normal cycle and one cycle with an extended pill-free interval of 10 days).[11] Investigators found that follicular growth up to preovulatory size was common in women missing the first one to three pills of the contraceptive cycle. The researchers noted, however, that normal ovulation did not occur when up to three pills were omitted.

Additional data come from a small, randomized trial of 15 women using a triphasic OC containing 35 µg EE and norethindrone.[12] The researchers found that the OC exerted a similar degree of pituitary and ovarian suppression even when the women missed four pills at varying times in the menstrual cycle (including when extending the pill-free interval from 7 to 11 days).

Given these data, the complex instructions about what to do in case of missing two pills may be unnecessary. In addition, simplified instructions eliminate the expense and inconvenience of backup contraception. No data exist, however, about the effect of missed pills on ovulation among women using the lowest estrogen OCs (20 µg EE), although Archer et al reported six of 18 pregnancies among women using a 20 µg EE OC occurred in women who had missed pills.[13] Even with low doses of estrogen, however, the progestin's effect on the cervical mucus should enhance contraceptive efficacy. Nonetheless, because the metabolism of sex steroids varies from woman to woman, the small possibility exists of escape ovulation in a woman who forgets two pills.

Clinicians should offer women written instructions about what to do if they miss pills in as simplified a format as possible. Patients should also have the phone number of an appropriate contact person to call in the event of missed pills, questions, or concerns about OCs. Women who have difficulty with missed pills should be offered more intensive counseling about how to take their pills correctly and given other options for contraception. Women who miss three or more OCs also should be evaluated for the need for emergency contraception.

Altering the Pill-Free Interval

Clinicians also may wish to alter the pill-free interval. Traditionally, the pill-free interval has consisted of 7 days of inactive placebo pills or no pills at all. Currently, many OC packages contain 28 pills: 21 active and seven placebo, with or without iron. One brand of combination OC alters the traditional 7-day hormone-free week. This OC contains 21 days of 20 µg EE plus 150 µg desogestrel, followed by 2 days of no hormone, and then 5 days of 10 µg estrogen for the remainder of the traditional pill-free week.

Clinicians have also altered OC regimens so that many active pills are taken without a break. Thus, 42, 63, or more active pills may be taken in a row without a break for withdrawal bleeding. This regimen may be helpful for women with particular medical disorders, including menstrual migraine, excessive uterine bleeding, or bleeding disorders.[14] (For further discussion, see the section on use of OCs to treat medical disorders.) Additionally,

Table 11

Summary of Instructions for Missed Pills from Combination OC Patient Package Inserts

Sunday Start Regimen

Consecutive Pills Omitted	Time of Cycle	Instruction
1	Any time	Take the missed pill as soon as remembered; take next one at scheduled time.
2	In the first 2 weeks	Take two a day (not at the same time) for 2 days, then resume schedule. Use backup contraception (condom, spermicide) for 7 days after missing pills.
2	In the third week of pills	Keep taking one pill daily until Sunday. Then, discard the rest of the pack and start a new pack immediately. Use backup contraception for 7 days after you missed pills.
3	Any time	Keep taking pills until Sunday. Discard the rest of the pack. Start a new pack immediately. The menses may not occur. Use backup contraception for 7 days after pills were missed.

Other than Sunday Start Regimens

Consecutive Pills Omitted	Time of Cycle	Instruction
1	Any time	Take the missed pill as soon as remembered; take next one at scheduled time.
2	In the first 2 weeks	Take two pills a day (not at the same time) for 2 days, then resume schedule. Use backup contraception for 7 days after missing pills.
2	In the third week of pills	Discard the rest of the pack. Start a new pack immediately. The menses may be skipped. Use backup contraception for 7 days after missing pills.
3	Any time	Discard the rest of the pack. Start a new pack immediately. The menses may be skipped. Use backup contraception for 7 days after missing pills.

Source: Goldzieher JW, 1998 (see reference 3). Used with permission.

55

Table 12

Guidelines for Missed Pills from Family Health International

- If a woman misses one active (hormone-containing) combination OC, she is not likely to become pregnant. When this happens, she should take the missed pill as soon as she remembers, then take the next pill at the regular time, even if this means she takes two pills in 1 day. No backup contraceptive method is necessary when one pill is missed.

- If a woman misses two or more active pills in a row, she should take an active pill daily for at least 7 consecutive days. During this time, she should abstain from sex or use a backup contraceptive (condom, spermicide).

- If her pill pack has fewer than seven active pills remaining, she should finish the remaining active pills and start a new pack immediately (without using inactive pills of the old pack or taking a 7-day break from pill taking). In this case, the woman will not have her menstrual bleeding at her regular time. If her pack has at least seven pills remaining, she should complete the pack and take her standard hormone-free break.

Source: Finger WR, 1996 (see reference 1).

some women without a menstrual-related disorder may prefer to experience withdrawal bleeding three or four times a year, rather than every month. Women can be reassured that this regimen has no adverse health effects. Continuous use of active pills can also provide OC users with the option of planning withdrawal bleeding so as not to experience bleeding during an inconvenient time (eg, on her wedding day). Shortening or eliminating the pill-free week may also provide the advantage of decreasing the possibility of escape ovulation.

Switching

Women who wish to stop using OCs and switch to another contraceptive can do so without having to finish the pill package. A woman can also switch to another brand of oral contraceptive at any time. However, because such side effects as breakthrough bleeding are likely to occur during the first 3 months, clinicians

Table 13

Simple Instructions for Missed Pills

If you miss one active (hormone-containing) pill—Take the forgotten pill as soon as it is remembered and the next one at the regular time.

If you miss two pills—Double up by taking two pills (not at the same time) each day for 2 days in a row. It is not necessary to use backup contraception (condom, spermicide) unless you are very worried about pregnancy. Ovulation and pregnancy are possible, but unlikely.

If you miss three or more active pills—Stop using your current package of OCs. Begin a new pack of pills (begin with the first active pill). Abstain from sex or use a backup method of contraception for 7 days. You may not have your menses this cycle—this is to be expected and not harmful. Continue taking the new package of pills as usual, one active pill every day until the hormone-free break. After withdrawal bleeding (your regular period), begin the next package of pills as usual.

should make every effort not to switch brands until at least a 3-month trial has been given. Switching OCs may lead to an increase in breakthrough bleeding and compliance problems.

Clinicians may want to counsel women who are changing from oral contraceptives to another method to start the new contraceptive method and then stop taking the OCs. This may decrease the chance of unintended pregnancy by providing overlapping protection.

Discontinuing OCs

Women may discontinue oral contraceptives at any time during the cycle; however, they should be counseled regarding the risk of unintended pregnancy and use of other methods of birth control. Unfortunately, many women discontinue using OCs because of side effects, fears about the pill, or failure to understand their risk of unintended pregnancy. Another reason given for discontinuation is breaking up with a partner and not needing contraception. Enhancing compliance is a critical counseling goal for clinicians involved in reproductive health. (For further discussion, see the section on improving successful use of OCs.)

Take Home Messages

- *Common routines for starting OCs include the Sunday start and the first-day start*

- *Another approach is the quick-start method, in which the woman begins the OC regimen on the day she receives her OC prescription, regardless of the day of the menstrual cycle*

- *Altering the pill-free interval can be convenient for women and helpful to treat excessive uterine bleeding or other medical disorders*

- *Women who are switching from OCs to another contraceptive method can be advised to start the new method before stopping OCs to decrease the chance of unintended pregnancy*

References

1. Finger WR. Oral contraceptives are safe, very effective. *Network* 1996;16:4-9.

2. Williams-Deane M, Potter LS. Current oral contraceptive use instructions: an analysis of patient package inserts. *Fam Plann Perspect* 1992;24:111-115.

3. Goldzieher JW. *Hormonal Contraception: Pills, Injections & Implants*. 4th ed. Ontario: EMIS-CANADA; 1998.

4. Fraser I, Jansen R. Why do inadvertent pregnancies occur in oral contraceptive users? Effectiveness of oral contraceptive regimens and interfering factors. *Contraception* 1983;27:531-551.

5. Molloy BG, Coulson KA, Lee JM, et al. "Missed pill" conception: fact or fiction? *BMJ* 1985;290:1474-1475.

6. Guillebaud J. The forgotten pill—and the paramount importance of the pill-free week. *Br J Fam Plann* 1987;12:35-43.

7. Hamilton CJCM, Hoogland HJ. Longitudinal ultrasonographic study of the ovarian suppressive activity of a low-dose triphasic oral contraceptive during correct and incorrect pill intake. *Am J Obstet Gynecol* 1989;161:1159-1162.

8. Killick SR. Ovarian follicles during oral contraceptive cycles: their potential for ovulation. *Fertil Steril* 1989;52:580-582.

9. Killick SR, Bancroft K, Oelbaum S, et al. Extending the duration of the pill-free interval during combined oral contraception. *Adv Contracept* 1990;6:33-40.

10. Landgren BM, Csemiczky G. The effect of follicular growth and luteal function of "missing the pill." A comparison between a monophasic and a triphasic combined oral contraceptive. *Contraception* 1991;43:149-159.

11. Elomaa K, Rolland R, Brosens I, et al. Omitting the first oral contraceptive pills of the cycle does not automatically lead to ovulation. *Am J Obstet Gynecol* 1998;179:41-46.

12. Letterie GS, Chow GE. Effect of "missed" pills on oral contraceptive effectiveness. *Obstet Gynecol* 1992;79:979-982.

13. Archer DF, Maheux R, DelConte A, et al. Efficacy and safety of a low-dose monophasic combination oral contraceptive containing 100 µg levonor-gestrel and 20 µg ethinyl estradiol (Alesse®). *Am J Obstet Gynecol* 1999;181: S39-S44.

14. Sulak PJ, Cressman BE, Waldrop E, et al. Extending the duration of active oral contraceptive pills to manage hormone withdrawal symptoms. *Obstet Gynecol* 1997;89:179-183.

1.10: 20 μg Estrogen OCs

Use of 20 μg estrogen oral contraceptives is growing. While these very low-dose OCs still occupy a small niche, the niche is expanding as more 20 μg pills enter the market (three since 1997). During the past decade, 20 μg OCs have been prescribed most frequently for women aged 40 years and older. The mean age of women using 20 μg pills has dropped recently, however, suggesting that clinicians are broadening their criteria for prescribing these oral contraceptives.

Relatively little is known about the safety and clinical performance of 20 μg pills compared with 30 and 35 μg estrogen OCs. Case-series reports (without comparison groups) of 20 μg pills have been performed.[1-7] Without a control group, however, these reports do not allow the clinician to compare these pills with others. Some investigations have compared formulations containing 20 μg EE and various progestins.[8-16] One head-to-head comparison indicates women using 20 μg OCs experience about half as much nausea, breast tenderness, and bloating as those using a 35 μg preparation. However, more extensive use of 20 μg pills will likely be required before their proposed benefits can be clearly defined.

Safety

Investigations of 20 μg estrogen OCs containing various progestins suggest a safety profile (adverse events and side effects) similar to that of 30 and 35 μg OCs.[1,2,6,7,16] No data, however, show 20 μg OCs to be safer than 30 or 35 μg estrogen pills.

Efficacy

Should efficacy be a concern when using very low-dose OCs? From Phase III clinical trials data, the FDA has concluded that combination OCs containing 20 μg estrogen effectively inhibit ovulation and are adequate for contraceptive control. For example, three studies of 20 μg EE in combination with desogestrel, gestodene, or levonorgestrel found some follicular development, but no ovulation, among women taking these preparations.[5,9,10] The first study compared two 20 μg pills containing either desogestrel or gestodene with a triphasic OC.[9] Among 51 women having 86 cycles monitored by ultrasonography, follicular-like structures were observed in nine women. The frequency of follicular growth was similar with all three OC preparations. No follicle progressed to >19 mm in diameter; a small amount of ovarian activity was present without ovulation.

The second investigation looked at ovarian activity during use of 20 μg EE in combination with 100 μg levonorgestrel.[5] Again, although some follicular activity was present, no escape ovulation occurred. The third study, comparing 20 μg EE preparations containing either desogestrel or gestodene, found similar results.[10]

Another study reported that a 20 μg preparation did not lead to more ovarian follicles or cysts compared with a 35 μg preparation.[17] Using vaginal ultrasonography, the researchers measured the size of ovarian follicles at baseline and during two treatment cycles in 63 women. The investigators found that only one woman had a follicle progress to an ovarian cyst of 35 mm in diameter. This woman took the 35 μg OC. No significant difference occurred in the number of women with follicles ≥10 mm in diameter between those taking 20 μg EE plus 150 μg desogestrel and those taking 35 μg EE plus 250 μg norgestimate. After 2 months of treatment, significantly fewer follicles occurred after two cycles compared to baseline (p<0.05).

One randomized, double-blind trial of 20 μg EE OCs containing either 500 μg norethisterone or 150 μg desogestrel found no ovulation among 118 women using these formulations.[14] In addition, the investigators found that the quality and quantity of the cervical mucus were minimal, and sonography indicated an endometrial thickness <8 mm in 85% to 90% of all cycles. The effects on cervical mucus and the endometrium presumably help to enhance contraceptive efficacy during use of these 20 μg OCs.

A group of European experts debated issues surrounding 20 μg pills in 1993.[18] The group concluded that 20 μg OCs appear to have the same level of effectiveness as 30 μg formulations, providing they are taken as prescribed. The group noted that individual variations in metabolism may narrow the margin of error with regard to forgotten pills and emphasized that clinicians educate women to improve compliance with the pill-taking regimen.

Side Effects

Cycle Control

The general pharmacological principle of using the lowest effective dose of a medication may collide—in the case of OCs—with cycle control and some noncontraceptive benefits. For example, one randomized controlled trial investigated the bioavailability of steroids and bleeding patterns and found decreasing cycle control with decreasing doses of both estrogen and progestin (although none contained 20 µg EE).[19]

Intermenstrual Bleeding

Studies of 20 µg OCs have generally found that breakthrough bleeding and spotting (intermenstrual bleeding) occur in about one-quarter to one-third of women in cycle 1 and diminish with time.[1,6,7,15] Studies comparing 20 µg EE formulations with gestodene or desogestrel have generally found comparable bleeding rates between preparations.[11,15] One investigation found intermenstrual bleeding (which included early withdrawal bleeding) in 45% of desogestrel users and 41% of gestodene users.[11] A few studies have found rates of intermenstrual bleeding (which included breakthrough bleeding, spotting, and early withdrawal bleeding) during cycle 1 ranging from 40% to 57%.[10,11,13,20]

Comparisons of formulations containing the same progestin and 20 or 30 µg EE have generally found that the lower-dose EE preparations have slightly higher rates of intermenstrual bleeding, although the differences between the groups have not always reached statistical significance.[8,21,22]

A comparison of 20 µg EE plus either 100 µg levonorgestrel or 1,000 µg norethindrone found significantly less intermenstrual bleeding for the levonorgestrel OC in cycles 2 and 3 (p<0.05).[13] In addition, the 20 µg EE formulation containing 100 µg levonorgestrel had similar cycle control to a triphasic norethindrone (500, 750, and 1,000 µg) preparation containing 35 µg EE.[12]

One head-to-head comparison has been performed comparing two 20 µg EE OCs containing the progestins desogestrel or levonorgestrel and a 35 µg preparation containing phased norgestimate.[16] Overall efficacy, safety, and cycle control among 463 OC-treated women were similar with all products; however, patients taking the 20 μg OCs reported significantly fewer (50% less) estrogen-related side effects (nausea, breast tenderness, bloating) compared to women using the 35 μg OC.

Amenorrhea

Studies of 20 μg OCs have found rates of amenorrhea ranging from 10% in cycle 1 to 2% in cycle 6,[1,2,6,7,11,15] although one study found 20% amenorrhea in cycle 1 with a 20 μg EE norethindrone preparation.[13] Generally, the rates of amenorrhea have been 5% or less.

Health Benefits

Little evidence exists regarding the effect of all low-dose pills (≤35 μg estrogen) on noncontraceptive health benefits. Data on health benefits were derived from older studies of higher-dose formulations. What data do exist suggest that the one health benefit that may be less—or missing—with low-dose formulations is the suppression of ovarian cyst development.

Early data indicated that high-dose OCs protected against the development of ovarian cysts.[23] Newer data suggest that the strength of the inhibition of ovarian cysts is attenuated or absent with lower-dose (30 to 35 μg EE) pills.[24,25] (For further discussion, see the section on health benefits of OCs.)

Ovarian and Endometrial Cancers

Will the reduction in estrogen dose to 20 μg affect the protection seen with higher-dose OCs (50 μg estrogen) against ovarian and endometrial cancers? Few data are available on lower-dose preparations (≤35 μg EE) and risk of ovarian cancer; however, if prevention of "incessant" ovulation or suppression of gonadotropins is the reason for the lower risk, then lower-dose pills could result in similar protection by preventing ovulation.

Use of high-dose OCs reduces the occurrence of endometrial cancer, a protection that increases with longer duration of use. The Cancer and Steroid Hormone Study found no significant difference in endometrial cancer protection between users of low- and high-dose OCs; however, this finding was based on very small numbers and no data were available on 20 μg OCs.[26]

Bone Mineral Density

Some evidence suggests that premenopausal use of OCs preserves bone mineral density; the data for 20 µg EE preparations, though, are sparse. A single investigation found that use of a 20 µg EE pill with desogestrel significantly increased vertebral bone density (p<0.001) in oligomenorrheic, perimenopausal women.[27]

Patient Populations

Whether some women will particularly benefit from use of 20 µg OCs is unknown. More large-scale clinical trials will be necessary to compare 20 µg formulations to those with 30 or 35 µg estrogen. Some data suggest that 20 µg estrogen OCs can be useful to minimize estrogen-related side effects.[16] Whether perimenopausal women may benefit from using the lowest effective dose of estrogen while still maintaining a regular hormonal pattern up to menopause has been suggested; however, no data exist to support or refute a benefit for older women.

Smokers

Some clinicians believe that women who smoke should use a lower EE formulation; however, no clinical data exist to show that use of a 20 µg EE pill is safer than a 30 or 35 µg pill in smokers. Clinicians should recommend that all women quit smoking.

Take Home Messages

- *Limited data exist on the safety, efficacy, and side effects of 20 µg OCs compared with 30 and 35 µg estrogen formulations*
- *Data indicate that 20 µg OCs effectively suppress ovulation*
- *Little is known about the effects of all low-dose pills (≤35 µg estrogen) on noncontraceptive health benefits*
- *Low-dose OCs (20 to 35 µg EE) may not suppress the development of ovarian cysts as effectively as higher-dose (≥50 µg EE) preparations*
- *Some data suggest that 20 µg estrogen OCs can be useful to minimize estrogen-related side effects*

References

1. The Mircette Study Group. An open label, multicenter, noncomparative safety and efficacy study of Mircette, a low-dose estrogen-progestin oral contraceptive. *Am J Obstet Gynecol* 1998;179:S2-S8.

2. Archer DF, Maheux R, DelConte A, et al. A new low-dose monophasic combination oral contraceptive (Alesse) with levonorgestrel 100 micrograms and ethinyl estradiol 20 micrograms. North American Levonorgestrel Study Group (NALSG). *Contraception* 1997;55:139-144.

3. Teichmann A, Martens H, Bordasch C, et al. The effects of a new low-dose combined oral contraceptive containing levonorgestrel on ovarian activity. *Eur J Contracept Reprod Health Care* 1996;1:245-256.

4. Trossarelli GF, Gennarelli G, Benedetto C, et al. Climacteric symptoms and control of the cycle in women aged 35 years or older taking an oral contraceptive with 0.150 mg desogestrel and 0.020 mg ethinylestradiol. *Contraception* 1995:51:13-18.

5. Spona J, Feichtinger W, Kindermann C, et al. Inhibition of ovulation by an oral contraceptive containing 100 µg levonorgestrel in combination with 20 µg ethinylestradiol. *Contraception* 1996;54:299-304.

6. Bannemerschult R, Hanker JP, Wunsch C, et al. A multicenter uncontrolled clinical investigation of the contraceptive efficacy, cycle control, and safety of a new low dose oral contraceptive containing 20 µg ethinyl estradiol and 100 µg levonorgestrel over six treatment cycles. *Contraception* 1997;56:285-290.

7. Archer DF, Maheux R, DelConte A, et al. Efficacy and safety of a low-dose monophasic combination oral contraceptive containing 100 µg levonorgestrel and 20 µg ethinyl estradiol (Alesse®). *Am J Obstet Gynecol* 1999;181: S39-S44.

8. Akerlund M, Rode A, Westergaard J. Comparative profiles of reliability, cycle control and side effects of two oral contraceptive formulations containing 150 µg desogestrel and either 30 µg or 20 µg ethinyl estradiol. *Br J Obstet Gynaecol* 1993;100:832-838.

9. Crosignani PG, Testa G, Vegetti W, et al. Ovarian activity during regular oral contraceptive use. *Contraception* 1996;54:271-273.

10. Fitzgerald C, Feichtinger W, Spona J, et al. A comparison of the effects of two monophasic, low-dose oral contraceptives on the inhibition of ovulation. *Adv Contracept* 1994;10:5-18.

11. Endrikat J, Jaques M-A, Mayerhofer M, et al. A twelve-month comparative clinical investigation of two low-dose oral contraceptives containing 20 µg ethinylestradiol/75 µg gestodene and 20 µg ethinylestradiol/150 µg desogestrel, with respect to efficacy, cycle control and tolerance. *Contraception* 1995; 52:229-235.

12. Reisman H, Martin D, Gast MJ. A multicenter randomized comparison of cycle control and laboratory findings with oral contraceptive agents containing 100 µg levonorgestrel with 20 µg ethinyl estradiol or triphasic norethindrone with ethinyl estradiol. *Am J Obstet Gynecol* 1999;181:S45-S52.

13. DelConte A, Loffer F, Grubb GS. Cycle control with oral contraceptives containing 20 micrograms of ethinyl estradiol. A multicenter, randomized comparison of levonorgestrel/ethinyl estradiol (100 micrograms/20 micrograms) and norethindrone/ethinyl estradiol (1000 micrograms/20 micrograms). *Contraception* 1999;59:187-193.

14. Rossmanith WG, Steffens D, Schramm G. A comparative randomized trial on the impact of two low-dose oral contraceptives on ovarian activity, cervical permeability, and endometrial receptivity. *Contraception* 1997;56:23-30.

15. Serfaty D, Vree ML. A comparison of the cycle control and tolerability of two ultra low-dose oral contraceptives containing 20 µg ethinyl estradiol and either 150 µg desogestrel or 75 µg gestodene. *Eur J Contracept Reprod Health Care* 1998;3:179-189.

16. Rosenberg MJ, Meyers A, Roy V. Efficacy, cycle control, and side effects of low- and lower-dose oral contraceptives: a randomized trial of 20 µg and 35 µg estrogen preparations. *Contraception* 2000;60:321-329.

17. Egarter C, Putz M, Strohmer H, et al. Ovarian function during low-dose oral contraceptive use. *Contraception* 1995;51:329-333.

18. Elstein M. Consensus paper. Low-dose contraceptive formulations: is further reduction in steroid dosage justified? *Adv Contracept* 1994;10:1-4.

19. Saleh WA, Burkman RT, Zacur HA, et al. A randomized trial of three oral contraceptives: comparison of bleeding patterns by contraceptive types and steroid levels. *Am J Obstet Gynecol* 1993;168:1740-1747.

20. Rosenberg MJ, Waugh MS, Higgins JE. The effect of desogestrel, gestodene, and other factors on spotting and bleeding. *Contraception* 1996;53:85-90.

21. Akerlund M. Clinical experience of a combined oral contraceptive with very low dose ethinyl estradiol. *Acta Obstet Gynecol Scand* 1997;76(suppl 164):63-65.

22. Teichmann AT, Schulte-Wintrop E, Lorkowski G. Theoretical and clinical basis for a further dose-reduction in levonorgestrel-containing oral contraceptives: discussion of results of clinical trials with LNG 100/EE 20. In: Teichmann AT, Corbin A, Elstein M, eds. *Levonorgestrel*. Stuttgart/New York: George Thieme Verlag; 1999:101-111.

23. Vessey M, Metcalfe A, Wells C, et al. Ovarian neoplasms, functional ovarian cysts, and oral contraceptives. *BMJ* 1987;294:1518-1520.

24. Lanes SF, Birmann B, Walker AM, et al. Oral contraceptive type and functional ovarian cysts. *Am J Obstet Gynecol* 1992;166:956-961.

25. Holt VL, Daling JR, McKnight B, et al. Functional ovarian cysts in relation to use of monophasic and triphasic oral contraceptives. *Obstet Gynecol* 1992;79:529-533.

26. The Cancer and Steroid Hormone Study of the Centers for Disease Control and the National Institute of Child Health and Human Development. Combination oral contraceptive use and the risk of endometrial cancer. *JAMA* 1987;257:796-800.

27. Gambacciani M, Spinetti A, Taponeco F, et al. Longitudinal evaluation of perimenopausal vertebral bone loss: effects of a low-dose oral contraceptive preparation on bone mineral density and metabolism. *Obstet Gynecol* 1994;83:392-396.

1.11: Side Effects

Today's low-dose oral contraceptives are very safe. The most recent evidence suggests that serious side effects, such as myocardial infarction and stroke, are rare and limited to women who smoke cigarettes or have hypertension or other cardiovascular risk factors. Among nonsmoking, otherwise healthy women, stroke and myocardial infarction are not associated with OC use. The risks associated with pregnancy generally far exceed the risks associated with OC use for most healthy reproductive age women.

Over the past 40 years, oral contraceptives have been studied extensively. Evidence concerning serious adverse effects of OCs was derived during a time when formulations contained much higher doses of steroids and when women were not screened to exclude those who smoked cigarettes or had hypertension. Newer studies indicate minimal risks associated with low-dose OCs. FDA-approved labeling, unfortunately, tends to be out of date. The FDA-approved package insert lists the following serious adverse effects associated with oral contraceptives:

- Stroke
- Myocardial infarction
- Venous thromboembolism
- Hypertension
- Gallbladder disease
- Liver tumors

On the other hand, a review of the latest evidence suggests the following are serious side effects of OCs:

1. An increased risk of cardiovascular events in women aged 35 years and older who smoke cigarettes;

2. A three- to fourfold increased risk of venous thromboembolism, which is less than that associated with pregnancy; and,

3. A substantially increased risk of venous thromboembolism among women using OCs who have clotting abnormalities, such as factor V Leiden.

Elevated Blood Pressure

An elevated blood pressure (most often minimal and still within the normal range) may occur in a small percentage of OC users;

however, the blood pressure usually returns to baseline when OCs are discontinued.

Gallbladder Disease and Liver Tumors

Evidence suggests that the risk of gallbladder disease may not be increased for women using low-dose preparations. Liver tumors, malignant or benign, are rare in healthy young women, regardless of whether they use OCs. Population-based data indicate no increased risk of liver cancer with OC use. (For further discussion, see the sections on OCs and gallbladder disease and liver cancer.)

Other Side Effects

Common benign side effects of OCs include such menstrual changes as intermenstrual or breakthrough bleeding, amenorrhea, and shortened or lighter menses. Early breakthrough bleeding and spotting are common, but usually subside after the first 3 months of OC use. (For further discussion, see the section on managing common side effects of OCs.)

Estrogen-related side effects include nausea, breast tenderness, and fluid retention. Subjective side effects, such as changes in mood, headaches, or an increase or decrease in libido, have been reported; however, they are difficult to assess. Skin changes, such as the hyperpigmentation of chloasma (mask of pregnancy), can also occur. The frequency of these side effects with low-dose OCs is low.

Unproven Side Effects

The FDA-approved package insert also lists many side effects that have been associated with OC use; however, evidence linking these side effects with OCs is lacking. Some of the questionable side effects are the following:

- Melanoma
- Hair loss
- Cataracts
- Intolerance to contact lenses
- Agitation
- Feelings of unrest/rejection
- Joint pain
- Respiratory infections
- Urinary tract problems
- Pneumonia
- Mouth sores
- Twitches

Alterations in Laboratory Values

Some laboratory values may be affected by combination OC use, particularly by the estrogen component. As doses of estrogen in OCs have decreased, however, so has the impact on laboratory values. Appendix A provides details concerning selected laboratory tests and the possible impact of OC use.

Take Home Messages

- *Serious adverse events are rare with use of low-dose OCs*

- *Myocardial infarction and stroke are not associated with low-dose OCs, provided the woman does not smoke cigarettes and is free of hypertension*

- *A three- to fourfold elevated risk of venous thromboembolism is associated with OC use; however, the risk is less than that associated with pregnancy*

- *An elevated blood pressure (most often minimal and within the normal range) may occur in a small percentage of OC users; however, the blood pressure usually returns to baseline when OCs are discontinued*

1.12: Approach to Common Side Effects

The approach to common oral contraceptive side effects most often consists of anticipatory guidance, careful history, and education of patients to dispel fears. Sometimes, diagnosis and management may involve an evaluation for STDs or switching to another formulation.

i. Cycle Control

Cycle control greatly affects the pill's acceptability to women. Breakthrough bleeding, spotting, and amenorrhea can be confusing or frightening. A woman may be concerned about whether the bleeding or spotting is her "real" period, if she should stop taking her OC, or if she has a medical problem (cancer or STDs). Unless thoroughly counseled as to the nature of breakthrough bleeding, women may stop taking the pill on their own—and about four-fifths either fail to use a substitute contraceptive or adopt one that is less effective.[1,2] Breakthrough bleeding is also a common cause for phone calls to the clinician's office.

Breakthrough Bleeding

Disruption of regular menstrual patterns can be disconcerting or frightening to patients or interfere with sexual relations.[3] OCs were designed with a 7-day hormone-free interval so that women would experience withdrawal bleeding in a pattern similar to menses. Cycle control with combination OCs is mediated by both the estrogen and progestin components. Manufacturers have experimented with altering the steroids in OCs in order to minimize breakthrough bleeding.

Breakthrough bleeding rates for most low-dose OCs vary from approximately 10% to 30% of women in the first month of use. Rates of breakthrough bleeding are similar for 20 µg OCs, although a few investigations have found rates of intermenstrual bleeding (which included breakthrough bleeding, spotting, and early withdrawal bleeding) during cycle 1 ranging from 40% to 57%.[4-7] (For further discussion, see the section on 20 µg OCs.)

A 1992 review of the literature by Rosenberg et al evaluated 25 studies of cycle control of various OCs.[8] These authors concluded that, in general, products containing norgestrel and levonorgestrel cause a lower incidence of spotting and breakthrough bleeding compared with norethindrone acetate and norethindrone, whether triphasic or monophasic (an effect which may be due to progestin pharmacokinetics).[9-14]

OCs containing the progestins desogestrel, gestodene (not available in the US), or norgestimate and 30 to 35 µg EE also provide acceptable cycle control.[15-20] No clear-cut differences among formulations have been documented, although a few studies have suggested that formulations containing gestodene may provide better cycle control than those containing desogestrel.[4,5,7,21] Cycle problems tend to lessen, however, within a few months of OC use, regardless of formulation. Limited data suggest that cycle control with 20 µg EE formulations is similar to that observed with 30 to 35 µg EE pills.[5-7,22-26]

A recent review of the literature[27] suggests that such factors as chlamydial infection, cigarette smoking, and missed pills may account for the differences found in the studies of OCs and breakthrough bleeding.[28-30] Studies of cycle control generally have had one or more of the following methodological problems:

- Large intra- and interstudy variations;
- Small sample size;
- Lack of control for such factors as age, cigarette smoking, and missed pills;
- Differences in study design and method analysis; and,
- Differences in the definitions of bleeding and spotting.

Amenorrhea

Women taking today's low-dose OC formulations experience amenorrhea infrequently (usually ≤5%); however, amenorrhea is important because women who miss a period may fear that something is wrong with them or, most commonly, that they are pregnant.

Management of Breakthrough Bleeding

The evaluation and management of patients who have irregular bleeding while taking oral contraceptives require thought and attention to the individual patient, rather than a standardized approach. One incorrect approach is to immediately suggest a different formulation of pills. This frequently results in the patient who states that she's tried "all" the different types of pills, yet has had breakthrough bleeding with all of them. When questioned further, she may report that she took each type for only a few days or weeks before being switched to a different type. Three cycles of a given OC are recommended to evaluate its effect.

Each patient who starts a new prescription for OC pills should be told that a minority of women will experience breakthrough bleeding during the first few months of use. If the patient does experience breakthrough bleeding, it is likely to resolve with time. Thus, the management of this side effect within the first 3 months of pill use consists simply of education and reassurance.

Clinicians should try not to change the pill formulation prior to 3 months of use unless it is clear that the patient is unwilling to continue the current preparation. Regardless of formulation prescribed, one cannot predict for an individual woman whether or not she will experience breakthrough bleeding.

The issue of pill compliance should be explored when a patient experiences breakthrough bleeding. Missed pills are so common that the clinician should always inquire about missed pills first in relationship to breakthrough bleeding. The problem can be circular: missed pills result in breakthrough bleeding, which leads to more dissatisfaction, which may lead to more missed pills (Figure 9). In addition, clinicians should consider chlamydial infection or pregnancy. Women who smoke should be counseled about the potential for increased breakthrough bleeding during OC use.

If breakthrough bleeding persists after 3 months of OC use, several management options are available. If the bleeding is slight, infrequent, and not bothersome, no treatment may be necessary. If the bleeding is bothersome, additional estrogen to stabilize the endometrium may be appropriate. One approach adds oral estrogens to the patient's current pill formulation (1.25 mg conjugated equine estrogen or its equivalent [eg, 0.02 mg ethinyl estradiol] daily for 1 week at the time the breakthrough bleeding occurs; repeated, if necessary).

Figure 9

Cycle of Breakthrough Bleeding, Missed Pills, and OC Dissatisfaction

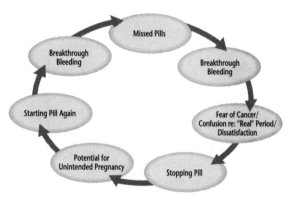

Other approaches used by some clinicians include:

- Doubling up on active pills for 2 to 3 days until the breakthrough bleeding stops, then resuming one active pill daily;

- Doubling up on active pills for the rest of the cycle;

- Providing a course of nonsteroidal anti-inflammatory medication; and,

- Changing to a continuous OC regimen.

Data indicate that nonsteroidal anti-inflammatory drug use may help alleviate breakthrough bleeding in women using implants, although no clinical trials document efficacy for OC users.[31]

Management of Amenorrhea

The management of amenorrhea consists of a pregnancy test and counseling. Clinicians should ask about missed pills and the possibility of pregnancy. If the patient has not been at risk of pregnancy, reassurance is appropriate.

Another management approach is to add a small dose of estrogen to the OC regimen in order to increase the thickness of the endometrium and improve the likelihood of withdrawal bleeding.

Take Home Messages

- *Cycle irregularity can lead to OC discontinuation*
- *In general, randomized controlled trials have shown that products containing levonorgestrel provide better cycle control than those containing norethindrone; few comparative data with desogestrel and norgestimate are available*
- *Several factors, however, limit conclusions that can be drawn from these studies:*
  - *Variations in individual metabolism*   *– Cigarette smoking*
  - *Presence of chlamydial infection*   *– Missed pills*
- *By the end of three cycles, rates of breakthrough bleeding are the same for almost all preparations; management of breakthrough bleeding includes reassurance*
- *Try not to switch formulations before 3 months of a given OC*
- *Additional estrogen supplementation may be warranted for patients in whom breakthrough bleeding is bothersome*
- *Reassure patients that breakthrough bleeding and amenorrhea can occur and are not harmful*

References

1. Rosenberg MJ, Waugh MS. Oral contraceptive discontinuation: a prospective evaluation of frequency and reasons. *Am J Obstet Gynecol* 1998;179:577-582.

2. Trussell J, Vaughan B. Contraceptive failure, method-related discontinuation, and resumption of use: results from the 1995 National Survey of Family Growth. *Fam Plann Perspect* 1999;31:64-72,93.

3. Hillard PJA. The patient's reaction to side effects of oral contraceptives. *Am J Obstet Gynecol* 1989;161:1412-1415.

4. Rosenberg MJ, Waugh MS, Higgins JE. The effect of desogestrel, gestodene, and other factors on spotting and bleeding. *Contraception* 1996;53:85-90.

5. Endrikat J, Jaques M-A, Mayerhofer M, et al. A twelve-month comparative clinical investigation of two low-dose oral contraceptives containing 20 μg ethinylestradiol/75 μg gestodene and 20 μg ethinylestradiol/150 μg desogestrel, with respect to efficacy, cycle control and tolerance. *Contraception* 1995; 52:229-235.

6. DelConte A, Loffer F, Grubb GS. Cycle control with oral contraceptives containing 20 micrograms of ethinyl estradiol. A multicenter, randomized comparison of levonorgestrel/ethinyl estradiol (100 micrograms/20 micrograms) and norethindrone/ethinyl estradiol (1000 micrograms/20 micrograms). *Contraception* 1999;59:187-193.

7. Fitzgerald C, Feichtinger W, Spona J, et al. A comparison of the effects of two monophasic, low-dose oral contraceptives on the inhibition of ovulation. *Adv Contracept* 1994;10:5-18.

8. Rosenberg MJ, Long SC. Oral contraceptives and cycle control: a critical review of the literature. *Adv Contraception* 1992;8(suppl 1):35-45.

9. Droegemueller W, Rao Katta L, Bright TG, et al. Triphasic randomized clinical trial: comparative frequency of intermenstrual bleeding. *Am J Obstet Gynecol* 1989;161:1407-1411.

10. Schilling LH, Bolding T, Chenault B, et al. Evaluation of the clinical performance of three triphasic oral contraceptives: a multicenter, randomized comparative trial. *Am J Obstet Gynecol* 1989;160:1264-1268.

11. Dunson TR, McLaurin VL, Israngkura B, et al. A comparative study of two low-dose combined oral contraceptives: results from a multicenter trial. *Contraception* 1993;48:109-119.

12. Anstee P, Kovacs GT. A prospective, randomized study comparing the clinical effects of a norethisterone and a levonorgestrel containing low-dose oestrogen oral contraceptive pills. *Aust NZ J Obstet Gynaecol* 1993;33:81-83.

13. Edgren RA, Nelson JH, Gordon RT, et al. Bleeding patterns with low-dose monophasic oral contraceptives. *Contraception* 1989;40:285-297.

14. Ramos R, Apelo R, Osteria T, et al. A comparative analysis of three different dose combinations of oral contraceptives. *Contraception* 1989;39:165-177.

15. Notelovitz M. Contraceptive efficacy and safety of a monophasic oral contraceptive containing 150 µg desogestrel and 30 µg ethinyl estradiol: United States clinical experience using a "Sunday start" approach. *Fertil Steril* 1995; 64:261-266.

16. Halbe HW, de Melo NR, Bahamondes L, et al. Efficacy and acceptability of two monophasic oral contraceptives containing ethinylestradiol and either desogestrel or gestodene. *Eur J Contracept Reprod Health Care* 1998;3:113-120.

17. Corson SL. Efficacy and clinical profile of a new oral contraceptive containing norgestimate. *Acta Obstet Gynecol Scand* 1990;152(suppl):25-31.

18. Andolsek KM. Cycle control with triphasic norgestimate and ethinyl estradiol, a new oral contraceptive agent. *Acta Obstet Gynecol Scand* 1992;71(suppl 156):22-26.

19. Gauthier A, Upmalis D, Dain MP. Clinical evaluation of a new triphasic oral contraceptive: norgestimate and ethinyl estradiol. *Acta Obstet Gynecol Scand* 1992;71(suppl 156):27-32.

20. Comparato MR, Yabur JA, Bajares M. Contraceptive efficacy and acceptability of a monophasic oral contraceptive containing 30 µg ethinyl estradiol and 150 µg desogestrel in Latin-American women. *Adv Contracept* 1998;14:15-26.

21. Christie T. A clinical overview of a new triphasic contraceptive containing gestodene. *Int J Fertil* 1989;34(suppl):40-49.

22. The Mircette Study Group. An open label, multicenter, noncomparative safety and efficacy study of Mircette, a low-dose estrogen-progestin oral contraceptive. *Am J Obstet Gynecol* 1998;179:S2-S8.

23. Bannemerschult R, Hanker JP, Wunsch C, et al. A multicenter, uncontrolled clinical investigation of the contraceptive efficacy, cycle control, and safety of a new low dose oral contraceptive containing 20 µg ethinyl estradiol and 100 µg levonorgestrel over six treatment cycles. *Contraception* 1997;56: 285-290.

24. Archer DF, Maheux R, DelConte A, et al. Efficacy and safety of a low-dose monophasic combination oral contraceptive containing 100 µg levonorgestrel and 20 µg ethinyl estradiol (Alesse®). *Am J Obstet Gynecol* 1999;181: S39-S44.

25. Serfaty D, Vree ML. A comparison of the cycle control and tolerability of two ultra low-dose oral contraceptives containing 20 μg ethinyl estradiol and either 150 μg desogestrel or 75 μg gestodene. *Eur J Contracept Reprod Health Care* 1998;3:179-189.

26. Rosenberg MJ, Meyers A, Roy V. Efficacy, cycle control, and side effects of low- and lower-dose oral contraceptives: a randomized trial of 20 μg and 35 μg estrogen preparations. *Contraception* 2000;60:321-329.

27. Thorneycroft IH. Cycle control with oral contraceptives: a review of the literature. *Am J Obstet Gynecol* 1999;180:S280-S287.

28. Bontis J, Vavilis D, Panidis D, et al. Detection of *Chlamydia trachomatis* in asymptomatic women: relationship to history, contraception, and cervicitis. *Adv Contracept* 1994;10:309-315.

29. Krettek JE, Arkin SI, Chaisilwattana P, et al. *Chlamydia trachomatis* in patients who used oral contraceptives and had intermenstrual spotting. *Obstet Gynecol* 1993;81:728-731.

30. Rosenberg MJ, Waugh MS, Stevens CM. Smoking and cycle control among oral contraceptive users. *Am J Obstet Gynecol* 1996;174:628-632.

31. Diaz S, Croxatto NB, Pavez M, et al. Clinical assessment of treatments for prolonged bleeding in users of Norplant implants. *Contraception* 1990;42:97-109.

ii. Weight Gain

The prospect of gaining weight because one uses birth control can be worrisome. Women are particularly vulnerable to media images that clearly present a slender body as the ideal. Given strong societal pressures to be thin, many women, if they believe oral contraceptives can make them gain weight, will reject the method without knowing the truth.

A study by Emans et al found that 45% of adolescents were very concerned about the possibility of weight gain while taking the pill.[1] Teens seen in a suburban private practice were significantly more concerned about weight gain than those seen in a hospital-based adolescent clinic (86% vs 32%, p=0.001). Although no statistically significant difference in weight gain occurred between noncompliant and compliant patients, noncompliant patients were more likely to have *perceived* that they had gained weight while taking oral contraceptives, even though actual weight was often unchanged.[1] A Canadian survey of almost 500 adolescents identified weight gain as the side effect most young women had heard about—51% reported having heard about weight gain.[2]

The evidence suggests, however, that low-dose OCs cause no net weight gain among women using OCs over 1 year compared to women using nonhormonal methods. One double-blind, placebo-controlled trial of *high-dose* pills (those containing ≥50 µg estrogen) found no difference in weight among OC users versus nonusers.[3]

Carpenter and Neinstein found that sexually active adolescents using OCs for 12 months were no more likely to gain weight than those using intrauterine devices (IUDs) or barrier contraception.[4] Several other investigations also found no net weight gain among OC users.[5,6] One investigation measured the daily weights of 128 women during four cycles of triphasic OC use.[7] The study confirmed the lack of association between OC use and weight gain. Although a small minority (7%) of women gained ≥6 pounds, the largest proportion of women (52%) remained within 2 pounds of their starting weight, while 72% had either no weight change or a loss (Figure 10).

Figure 10

Mean Weight Change from Baseline among 128 Women Taking a Triphasic* Oral Contraceptive

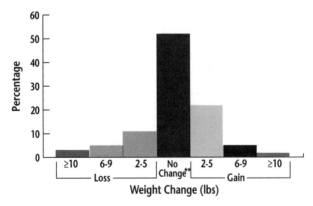

* 35 µg ethinyl estradiol and phased norethindrone
** Gain or loss of <2 lbs

Source: Rosenberg M, 1998 (see reference 7).

Management of Weight Gain

The management of weight gain consists of uncovering fears and reassuring patients that most patients using OCs will not gain weight. Women should be counseled about healthy eating habits and exercise and told that their weight will be checked during each visit.

Take Home Messages

- *As many women lose as gain weight while taking OCs; the majority have no change in weight*

- *Among adolescents, even the perception of weight gain is enough to negatively affect compliance—counsel patients about the facts*

- *Weigh the patient at each visit*

- *Counsel patients about healthy eating habits and exercise*

References

1. Emans SJ, Grace E, Woods ER, et al. Adolescents' compliance with the use of oral contraceptives. *JAMA* 1987;257:3377-3381.

2. Herold ES, Goodwin MS. Perceived side effects of oral contraceptives among adolescent girls. *Can Med Assoc J* 1980;123:1022-1026.

3. Goldzieher JW, Moses LE, Averkin E, et al. A placebo-controlled double-blind crossover investigation of the side effects attributed to oral contraceptives. *Fertil Steril* 1971;22:609-623.

4. Carpenter S, Neinstein LS. Weight gain in adolescent and young adult oral contraceptive users. *J Adolesc Health Care* 1986;7:342-344.

5. Reubinoff BE, Grubstein A, Meirow D, et al. Effects of low-dose estrogen oral contraceptives on weight, body composition, and fat distribution in young women. *Fertil Steril* 1995;63:516-521.

6. Moore L, Valuck R, McDougall C, et al. A comparative study of one-year weight gain among users of medroxyprogesterone acetate, levonorgestrel implants, and oral contraceptives. *Contraception* 1995;52:215-220.

7. Rosenberg M. Weight change with oral contraceptive use and during the menstrual cycle. Results of daily measurements. *Contraception* 1998;58:345-349.

iii. Nausea/Breast Tenderness/Fluid Retention

Nausea, breast tenderness, and fluid retention (bloating) are mediated by the estrogen component in OCs. Older, higher-dose preparations were more likely to be associated with these side effects than today's low-dose formulations.

Nausea is caused by estrogen in a dose-dependent fashion. Early trials found that nausea is self-limiting and generally disappears by the second or third cycle of high-dose OC use.[1] Other side effects mediated by excess estrogen include breast tenderness and fluid retention, which also are self-limiting and usually disappear within the first three cycles.

Management of nausea consists of counseling the patient that the side effect will likely disappear within 3 months. Other options include advising the patient to take the birth control pill at bedtime. Another possibility is to use the lowest-dose estrogen OC available, as some data indicate 20 µg OCs can cause 50% fewer estrogen-related side effects than a 35 µg OC.[2] If the nausea remains bothersome, an antiemetic can be prescribed. Management of breast tenderness and fluid retention also consists of reassuring the patient that these side effects are likely to diminish with time. Rarely, a mild diuretic can be used for a brief interval.

Take Home Messages

- *Nausea is caused by estrogen in a dose-dependent fashion*
- *Nausea, breast tenderness, and fluid retention can occur within the first 3 months of use; however, these side effects are less common with use of modern low-dose OCs*
- *Management of breast tenderness and fluid retention consists mainly of reassuring the patient and encouraging her to wait out 3 cycles of use*
- *Using the lowest estrogen OC formulation may reduce these side effects*

References

1. Hines DC, Goldzieher JW. Large-scale study of an oral contraceptive. *Fertil Steril* 1968;19:841-866.

2. Rosenberg MJ, Meyers A, Roy V. Efficacy, cycle control, and side effects of low- and lower-dose oral contraceptives: a randomized trial of 20 µg and 35 µg estrogen preparations. *Contraception* 2000;60:321-329.

iv. Libido/Mood Changes/Depression

Women using high-dose oral contraceptives reported changes in libido; however, OCs have no clear effect on sex drive. In addition, depression and mood changes were reported by women using high-dose OCs. The incidence of these side effects is infrequent (generally ≤5%), however, with low-dose OCs.

Early studies reported various changes in libido (increase, decrease, or no effect) with OC use. These early studies suffer from methodologic difficulties, however. For example, the studies generally did not assess sexual activity prior to OC use and the term *libido* was generally undefined. Women should be counseled that there is no clear effect of oral contraceptives on sex drive.

Mood changes, particularly depression, were first reported in 1963. Some early studies of women using high-dose pills observed an improved mood while others noted depression or no effect.[1-3] The rates of depression varied from 10% to 56% of women using OCs. At first, concern regarding depression seemed biologically plausible because biochemical studies found deficiencies in urinary tryptophan and pyridoxine metabolites. Eventually, however, this biochemical pathway was ruled out as a causal relationship for linking OCs to depression. Current studies suggest little or no effect of low-dose OCs on mood changes and depression.[4-6]

Take Home Messages

- *Women infrequently report changes in libido with low-dose OC use; women who report changes in libido can be reassured that OCs have no known effect on sex drive*

- *Mood changes and depression were reported among women using high-dose OCs; however, a causal link to these subjective complaints could not be found*

- *Today's low-dose OCs are infrequently associated with mood changes*

References

1. Slap GB. Oral contraceptives and depression: impact, prevalence and cause. *J Adolesc Health Care* 1981;2:53-64.

2. Glick ID. Mood and behavioral changes associated with the use of the oral contraceptive agents. A review of the literature. *Psychopharmacol* 1967;10: 363-374.

3. Keefe D. Nervous system. In: Goldzieher JW, Fotherby K, eds. *Pharmacology of the Contraceptive Steroids*. New York: Raven Press; 1994:283-298.

4. Vessey MP, McPherson K, Lawless M, et al. Oral contraception and serious psychiatric illness: absence of an association. *Br J Psychiatry* 1985;146:45-49.

5. The Mircette Study Group. An open label, multicenter, noncomparative safety and efficacy study of Mircette, a low-dose estrogen-progestin oral contraceptive. *Am J Obstet Gynecol* 1998;179:S2-S8.

6. Archer DF, Maheux R, DelConte A, et al. A new low-dose monophasic combination oral contraceptive (Alesse) with levonorgestrel 100 micrograms and ethinyl estradiol 20 micrograms. North American Levonorgestrel Study Group (NALSG). *Contraception* 1997;55:139-144.

1.13: Return to Fertility

The evidence is clear that modern oral contraceptives do not cause permanent infertility.[1-3] Despite the medical evidence, women may fear that oral contraceptives can cause permanent damage to their reproductive system. Women may also hold mistaken beliefs about how OCs affect their fertility. For example, patients may not realize that once they stop taking OCs, fertility returns quickly. They may incorrectly believe the contraceptive effect will last for a few months.

A recent analysis of the Nurses' Health Study II found no significant overall reduction in fertility in women using OCs.[4] The researchers based their findings on a nested case-control study within a cohort of about 116,000 female nurses. Almost 90% of women reported an eventual pregnancy, suggesting that absolute fertility was not impaired.

Many women, although not all, will ovulate in the month following discontinuation. Women who choose to discontinue OCs should be advised to use another method of birth control if they do not wish to become pregnant.

Women who wish to become pregnant, however, should be told that they may experience a temporary delay in conception. Many studies have found a temporary delay in conception after use of OCs,[1-3] although some evidence suggest the delay is shorter with modern low-dose formulations compared to higher-dose formulations.[5]

A 1990 study by Bracken et al suggests that delayed conception occurs in pill users significantly more frequently than in nonusers and that high-dose OCs delay conception more than low-dose OCs.[5] The study was conducted over 25 months and evaluated 248 former OC users and 1,365 women who discontinued using other methods, such as the diaphragm, spermicide, or IUD. The mean time for nonusers to conceive was 3.6 cycles; low-dose pill users took a mean 4.0 cycles to conceive; high-dose (≥ 50 µg estrogen) pill users took a mean of 4.8 cycles to conceive (p=0.05 for low- compared to high-dose users). Because a dose-related effect appeared, the investigators concluded that OC use was responsible for the fertility delays.

A retrospective analysis by Harlap and Baras compared women stopping the pill in order to conceive with women stopping other methods.[6] Women who had used high-dose OCs were 30% less likely to have conceived in the first month after stopping the pill than women who had stopped other nonhormonal methods. This discrepancy disappeared, however, by the third month.

Women need to understand that a delay in conception may occur after discontinuing the pill. They should be reassured, however, that the delay is temporary and that previous fertility levels usually return within 3 to 12 months.

Take Home Messages

- OCs do not cause permanent infertility
- Fertility returns quickly after stopping OCs, although fertility rates are slightly lower during the first 3 to 12 months as compared to women discontinuing nonhormonal methods
- Data suggest low-dose OCs cause less of a delay to conception than high-dose OCs

---

References

1. Vessey MP, Wright NH, McPherson K, et al. Fertility after stopping different methods of contraception. *BMJ* 1978;1:265-267.

2. Linn S, Schoenbaum SC, Monson RR, et al. Delay in conception for former 'pill' users. *JAMA* 1982;247:629-632.

3. Fraser IS, Weisberg E. Fertility following discontinuation of different methods of fertility control. *Contraception* 1982;26:389-415.

4. Chasen-Taber L, Willett WC, Stampfer MJ, et al. Oral contraceptives and ovulatory causes of delayed fertility. *Am J Epidemiol* 1997;146:258-265.

5. Bracken MB, Hellenbrand KG, Holford TR. Conception delay after oral contraceptive use: the effect of estrogen dose. *Fertil Steril* 1990;53:21-27.

6. Harlap S, Baras M. Conception-waits in fertile women after stopping oral contraceptives. *Int J Fertil* 1984;29:73-80.

2.1: Metabolic Effects

*Concerns about potential adverse metabolic effects of oral
contraceptives have traditionally centered on carbohydrate
and lipid metabolism. After numerous studies of these issues,
however, the results suggest changes in these metabolic processes
have little or no relevance to clinical practice.*

i. Carbohydrate Metabolism/Diabetes

*Studies indicate that the majority of healthy women, those with a
history of gestational diabetes, and those with insulin-dependent
diabetes may safely use OCs. Importantly, modern low-dose OCs have
less impact than older formulations on carbohydrate metabolism, as this
effect is mediated by the progestin and is dose dependent. In insulin-
dependent diabetic women, a careful risk-to-benefit assessment
is especially warranted because pregnancy carries risks for both mother
and fetus.*

Glucose Tolerance in Healthy Women

Several large, prospective studies have found that OCs do not
increase a woman's chance of developing diabetes mellitus.[1,2] The
initial report from the Royal College of General Practitioners'
(RCGP) Oral Contraception Study and the Oxford Family Planning
Association Study found no difference in the occurrence of diabetes
mellitus among current users, past users, and women who never
used the pill.[1] These findings were based on over 317,000 woman-
years of observation.

The latest findings from the RCGP confirm previous results.[3]
Based on almost 106,000 woman-years of current OC use and
almost 175,000 woman-years of former OC use, the researchers
found no evidence of an increased risk of developing diabetes
mellitus among current users (RR=0.8; 95% CI, 0.5-1.3). This was
true even for long durations of use (10 years or more). Former pill
use also conferred no additional risk (RR=0.8; 95% CI, 0.6-1.1).

The Nurses' Health Study also found no increased risk of non-
insulin-dependent (type 2) diabetes mellitus in current or former

OC users.[4] The Nurses' Health Study is a large, prospective cohort survey that has followed almost 122,000 female nurses since 1976. During over 1 million person-years of follow-up, 2,276 women were diagnosed with type 2 diabetes. Among these women, current users had no increased risk of type 2 diabetes mellitus (RR=0.9; 95% CI, 0.5-1.6) when compared to women who had never used OCs. In addition, former users of the pill also had no increased risk (RR=1.1; 95% CI, 1.0-1.2). The investigators found no difference in risk after a multivariate adjustment for age, body mass index, family history of diabetes, cigarette smoking, menopause, and postmenopausal hormone use. The Walnut Creek Contraceptive Drug Study also found no evidence that high-dose OCs led to impaired glucose tolerance or diabetes.[5]

Prior Gestational Diabetes

Women with prior gestational diabetes also do not appear at increased risk of developing diabetes mellitus from use of OCs. Kjos and colleagues studied 230 women with previously diagnosed gestational diabetes who used low-dose OCs for up to 13 months of treatment.[6] The researchers randomly assigned patients to use an OC containing either ethinyl estradiol plus norethindrone or EE plus levonorgestrel. A 75 g, 2-hour glucose tolerance test and fasting lipid profile were performed at entry, after 3 months, and after 6 to 13 months of treatment. The class of gestational diabetes appeared to have the most profound impact on deterioration in glucose tolerance rather than use of oral contraceptives.

A large, retrospective cohort study of 904 Latina women with previous gestational diabetes mellitus found similar results.[7] Women using low-dose combination OCs had no increased risk of developing diabetes compared with those using nonhormonal contraception. The 3-year cumulative incidence rate of diabetes in combination OC users was 25% vs 27% in women using nonhormonal contraception. The researchers found no evidence of an accelerated rate of diabetes for up to 5 years of continuous use of OCs. Women used OC preparations containing the progestins norethindrone or levonorgestrel; no differences were found between these groups.

Diabetes Mellitus

Two recent studies also suggest that OCs do not enhance the progression of diabetes.[8,9] Klein et al assessed data from the population-based Wisconsin Epidemiologic Study of Diabetic Retinopathy.[8] Among approximately 1,000 women, 384 reported a history of OC use. The researchers found that neither current or past use nor number of years of OC use was associated with severity of retinopathy.

Garg et al followed almost 300 young women with diabetes mellitus.[9] In this retrospective cohort study at a university hospital diabetes clinic, 43 diabetic women who had used OCs for 1 year or longer were compared with a control group of 43 diabetic women who had never used OCs. The final mean albumin excretion rates, reflecting diabetic renal damage, and the mean eye grades were not significantly different between the groups. The finding suggests that OC use does not pose an additional risk for the development of early diabetic retinopathy or nephropathy when used by young women with insulin-dependent diabetes mellitus.

OC Formulations

The differences among low-dose OC formulations are also minimal.[10,11] van der Vange and colleagues performed a comparative study of seven currently used low-dose combination OCs.[10] They examined OCs containing 30 to 40 µg EE and various progestins, including norethindrone, desogestrel, levonorgestrel, cyproterone acetate (not available in the US), and gestodene (also not available). The area under the curve for insulin and glucose did not change during treatment with any of the preparations, and the researchers inferred that none of these OCs had any adverse effect on glucose metabolism after 6 months.

Weighing the Risk-to-Benefit Ratio

For healthy women, combination OCs pose no additional risk of diabetes; this also appears to be true for women with previous gestational diabetes. For the insulin-dependent diabetic woman, OCs may be used when the patient has made an informed decision based on her current diabetic status and her unwillingness to use other methods. Clinicians should carefully weigh the benefits versus the risks of OC use for diabetic women, in whom pregnancy carries a risk of progression of retinopathy, nephropathy, coronary heart disease, and congenital malformations. A careful assessment needs to be made of the risk-to-benefit ratio for various contraceptives when considering their use among women with medical disorders.[12]

Among diabetics, the use of a highly effective birth control method should be encouraged. Pregnancy may then be planned during a time of optimal glycemic control. WHO medical eligibility criteria suggest caution or no combination OC use among diabetic women with vascular complications or diabetes of >20 years' duration. These cautions are based on theoretical concerns about the potential increased risk of cardiovascular disease and thrombosis; however, no data exist to support these recommendations. (For further discussion, see the section on medical eligibility criteria for OC use.) Although no evidence shows that OCs hasten the progression of cardiovascular complications in diabetic women, many clinicians recommend the IUD or progestin-only methods for diabetic women with peripheral vascular or coronary artery disease.

Take Home Messages

- *Large epidemiologic studies show no increased risk of diabetes among women using OCs*

- *Women with prior gestational diabetes do not appear at increased risk of future diabetes due to OC use*

- *Some evidence suggests OC use does not enhance the progression of either diabetic retinopathy or nephropathy among women with insulin-dependent diabetes*

- *OCs have not been shown to accelerate the progression of diabetic cardiovascular complications*

- *No significant difference in carbohydrate metabolism exists among various OC formulations*

- *The risk-to-benefit ratio of OC use in diabetic women needs to be carefully assessed, as pregnancy carries potentially serious consequences for mother and fetus*

References

1. Wingrave SJ, Kay CR, Vessey MP. Oral contraceptives and diabetes mellitus. *BMJ* 1979;1:23.

2. Russell-Briefel R, Ezzati TM, Perlman JA, et al. Impaired glucose tolerance in women using oral contraceptives: United States, 1976-1980. *J Chron Dis* 1987;40:3-11.

3. Hannaford PC, Kay CR. Oral contraceptives and diabetes mellitus. *BMJ* 1989; 299:1315-1316.

4. Rimm EB, Manson JE, Stampfer MJ, et al. Oral contraceptive use and the risk of type 2 (non-insulin-dependent) diabetes mellitus in a large prospective study of women. *Diabetologia* 1992;35:967-972.

5. Duffy TJ, Ray R. Oral contraceptive use: prospective follow-up of women with suspected glucose intolerance. *Contraception* 1984;30:197-208.

6. Kjos SL, Shoupe D, Douyan S, et al. Effect of low-dose oral contraceptives on carbohydrate and lipid metabolism in women with recent gestational diabetes: results of a controlled, randomized, prospective study. *Am J Obstet Gynecol* 1990:163:1822-1827.

7. Kjos SL, Peters RK, Xiang A, et al. Contraception and the risk of type 2 diabetes mellitus in Latina women with prior gestational diabetes mellitus. *JAMA* 1998;280:533-538.

8. Klein BEK, Moss SE, Klein R. Oral contraceptives in women with diabetes. *Diabetes Care* 1990;13:895-898.

9. Garg SK, Chase HP, Marshall G, et al. Oral contraceptives and renal and retinal complications in young women with insulin-dependent diabetes mellitus. *JAMA* 1994;271:1099-1102.

10. van der Vange N, Kloosterboer HJ, Haspels AA. Effect of seven low-dose combined oral contraceptive preparations on carbohydrate metabolism. *Am J Obstet Gynecol* 1987;156:918-922.

11. Simon D, Senan C, Garnier P, et al. Effects of oral contraceptives on carbohydrate and lipid metabolism in a healthy population: The Telecom Study. *Am J Obstet Gynecol* 1990;163:382-387.

12. Jones KP, Wild RA. Contraception for patients with psychiatric or medical disorders. *Am J Obstet Gynecol* 1994;170:1575-1580.

ii. Lipid Metabolism/Atherogenesis

Are changes in the lipid profile induced by oral contraceptives relevant to clinical practice? The evidence suggests they are not, although some researchers have theorized that alterations in low-density lipoprotein and high-density lipoprotein profiles may influence long-term risk of coronary atherosclerosis in women using OCs. Data on the long-term effects of OC use in women and experimental animals do not support this concept.

Cardiovascular disease in women taking oral contraceptives is primarily thrombotic, rather than atherogenic, and is attributed to the estrogen component. Although researchers have performed numerous studies comparing lipoprotein subfraction changes among various OC formulations, most differences are minor and remain within normal limits, and their relevance to clinical practice is questionable.[1]

If alterations in lipids induced by OCs did cause an increased risk of atherogenesis, then an increased risk of disease should be seen in women who used OCs, especially for long durations. No such association is evident. Analyses of the Nurses' Health Study found no increased risk of subsequent cardiovascular disease among former OC users, even with prolonged previous use.[2-4] In fact, in one study of premenopausal women who had had a myocardial infarction, typical diffuse coronary atherogenesis was found less frequently in OC users.[5]

Data from cynomolgus macaque monkeys also do not support the notion that OCs increase the risk of atherogenic plaque formation.[6-9] These monkeys serve as an important atherogenesis research model for several reasons:

1. The histology of macaque coronary atheromas is identical to that of humans;

2. The female monkeys' reproductive physiology is similar to human females; and,

3. Their lipid profile and its response to OCs are also similar to humans.

Studies using this animal model suggest that the estrogenic effect of OCs may help to prevent atherosclerosis.[8] Researchers compared the effects of two contraceptive preparations on diet-induced atherosclerosis in female macaques. One formulation contained EE plus norgestrel, the other contained EE plus ethynodiol diacetate (which metabolizes to norethindrone). The dose given to the animals was adjusted to be comparable to that given to women during high-dose OC treatment.

The OCs prevented plaque formation despite adverse lipoprotein profiles. Based on plasma lipoprotein measurements, the predicted amount of coronary artery atherosclerosis among the OC groups should have been 1.3 to 2.7 times greater than that seen in the control animals. Instead, coronary atherosclerosis among the OC groups was reduced by 55% to 83%. This apparent paradox indicated a large protective effect of OC treatment with respect to coronary artery atherosclerosis despite the adverse lipoprotein profile induced by the OCs.[8]

The type of progestin given in low-dose combination OCs also appears to be unrelated to the later development of atherogenic cardiovascular disease. Both estranes (norethindrone) and gonanes (levonorgestrel, desogestrel, gestodene, and norgestimate) have a similar and clinically unimportant impact on lipids.[10,11]

Take Home Messages

- *Cardiovascular complications in women using OCs are not atherogenic in origin*

- *Data from the Nurses' Health Study indicate no increased risk of subsequent cardiovascular disease among former OC users*

- *Data from cynomolgus macaque monkeys, an accepted animal model for atherogenesis, suggest that the estrogen in OCs protects against the development of atherosclerosis*

- *Lipid values among OC users tend to vary only within the normal range*

- *The progestins used in low-dose combination OCs and their effect on lipids appear irrelevant for the later development of coronary atherogenesis*

References

1. Hoppe G. The clinical relevance of oral contraceptive pill-induced plasma lipid changes: facts and fiction. *Am J Obstet Gynecol* 1990;163:388-391.

2. Colditz GA and The Nurses' Health Study Research Group. Oral contraceptive use and mortality during 12 years of follow-up: the Nurses' Health Study. *Ann Intern Med* 1994;120:821-826.

3. Stampfer MJ, Willett WC, Colditz GA, et al. A prospective study of past use of oral contraceptive agents and risk of cardiovascular diseases. *N Engl J Med* 1988;319:1313-1317.

4. Stampfer MJ, Willett WC, Colditz GA, et al. Past use of oral contraceptives and cardiovascular disease: a meta-analysis in the context of the Nurses' Health Study. *Am J Obstet Gynecol* 1990;163:285-291.

5. Engel HJ, Engel E, Lichtlen PR. Coronary atherosclerosis and myocardial infarction in young women—role of oral contraceptives. *Eur Heart J* 1983; 4:1-8.

6. Adams MR, Clarkson TB, Koritnik DR, et al. Contraceptive steroids and coronary artery atherosclerosis in cynomolgus macaques. *Fertil Steril* 1987; 47:1010-1018.

7.   Clarkson TB, Adams MR, Kaplan JR, et al. From menarche to menopause: coronary artery atherosclerosis and protection in cynomolgus monkeys. *Am J Obstet Gynecol* 1989;160:1280-1285.

8.   Clarkson TB, Shively CA, Morgan TM, et al. Oral contraceptives and coronary artery atherosclerosis of cynomolgus monkeys. *Obstet Gynecol* 1990;75:217-222.

9.   Adams MR, Kaplan JR, Manuck SB, et al. Inhibition of coronary artery atherosclerosis by 17-beta estradiol in ovariectomized monkeys. Lack of an effect of added progesterone. *Arteriosclerosis* 1990;10:1051-1057.

10. Patsch W, Brown SA, Gotto AM, et al. The effect of triphasic oral contraceptives on plasma lipids and lipoproteins. *Am J Obstet Gynecol* 1989;161:1396-1401.

11. Notelovitz M, Feldman E, Gillespy M, et al. Lipid and lipoprotein changes in women taking low-dose, triphasic oral contraceptives: a controlled, comparative, 12-month clinical trial. *Am J Obstet Gynecol* 1989;160:1037-1048.

2.2: Cardiovascular Disease

Elevated blood pressure with low-dose OC use is uncommon, but does occur in a small minority of women. Modern, low-dose oral contraceptives, when used by nonsmoking, normotensive women, are not associated with myocardial infarction (MI) or stroke. OCs are associated with about a three- to fourfold increased risk of venous thromboembolism (VTE), although the risk is substantially less than that associated with pregnancy.

i. Elevated Blood Pressure

Modern low-dose oral contraceptives induce no change or minimal changes in blood pressure. The benefits of using OCs may outweigh the risks for a woman with borderline or mild hypertension, as well, as long as the woman can be treated appropriately and have her blood pressure monitored regularly.

High-Dose OCs

High-dose OCs were found to cause elevated blood pressure in some studies, but not others. For example, a WHO prospective trial of 1,400 women using either high-dose OCs (≥ 50 µg EE) or an IUD found small changes in systolic and diastolic blood pressures.[1] The rise in systolic blood pressure was 4 to 5 mmHg higher for OC users compared to women using IUDs, while the diastolic pressures were 2 to 3 mmHg higher.

On the other hand, researchers found no significant effect of high-dose OC use on mean arterial blood pressure among almost 2,700 black women attending a large southeastern family planning clinic.[2] The women, considered high risk because of their ethnic background, had their blood pressures monitored periodically for 6 to 24 months.

Low-Dose OCs

Evidence concerning blood pressure and low-dose OCs suggests the effects are minimal. Elevated blood pressure, if it occurs, most often remains within the normal range and usually returns to baseline after stopping OCs. A recent analysis from the Nurses'

Health Study II suggested that only about 42 cases of elevated blood pressure occurred per 10,000 person-years in women using current low-dose pill formulations.[3] A randomized trial of 131 women using four different OCs with various progestins and 30 µg EE found only small increases in systolic and diastolic pressures, no matter which formulation was used.[4] A trial of 61 high-risk women (those with a previous history of hypertension) and 61 low-risk women using low-dose OCs found that mean systolic and diastolic pressures of the high-risk women did not rise when compared with their own baseline blood pressure.[5]

Women with a history of hypertension may use OCs as long as their blood pressure can be monitored regularly. Because hypertension is an independent risk factor for stroke and MI, women with borderline or mild hypertension should probably use OCs only if their blood pressure can be treated and monitored regularly.

Take Home Messages

- *Modern low-dose OCs have little or no effect on blood pressure*

- *The Nurses' Health Study II found only 42 cases per 10,000 person-years of elevated blood pressure among low-dose OC users*

- *The benefits of OCs may outweigh the risks for women with borderline or mild hypertension as long as the elevated blood pressure can be treated and monitored*

- *Progestin-only OCs may be used by women with hypertension*

References

1.   WHO Task Force on Oral Contraceptives. The WHO multicentre trial of the vasopressor effects of combined oral contraceptives. 1. Comparisons with IUD. *Contraception* 1989;40:129-145.

2.   Blumenstein BA, Douglas MB, Hall WD. Blood pressure changes and oral contraceptive use: a study of 2,676 black women in the southeastern United States. *Am J Epidemiol* 1980;112:539-552.

3.   Chasan-Taber L, Willett WC, Manson JE, et al. Prospective study of oral contraceptives and hypertension among women in the United States. *Circulation* 1996;94:483-489.

4. Nichols M, Robinson G, Bounds W, et al. Effect of four combined oral contraceptives on blood pressure in the pill-free interval. *Contraception* 1993;47:367-376.

5. Tsai CC, Williamson HO, Kirkland BH, et al. Low-dose oral contraception and blood pressure in women with a past history of elevated blood pressure. *Am J Obstet Gynecol* 1985;151:28-32.

ii. Stroke

The most recent evidence confirms the safety of low-dose oral contra-ceptives with regard to stroke. Over the past 2 decades, estimates of the magnitude of the risk for stroke have dropped, probably due to changes in pill formulation, prescribing practices, and use of more sophisticated epi-demiologic methods. In addition, diagnostic accuracy has improved. Most importantly, new OC users are now screened for cigarette smoking and hypertension, both independent risk factors for stroke and major con-founders of early studies.

Two studies published in 1996 provide valuable new data on stroke and OC use. The first, from Petitti et al, examined users of OCs in a large health maintenance organization (HMO) in Califor-nia.[1] The second, from the World Health Organization, studied OC users in Europe and developing countries.[2,3]

Evidence from the United States

Petitti et al provide the first evaluation of US data on the relation between current, lower-dose OC use and the risk of stroke. This large, population-based, case-control study concluded that stroke is rare among women of childbearing age and that low-estrogen OC use does not appear to affect the risk of stroke in healthy women.[1]

The study population came from the Kaiser Permanente Medical Care Programs of Northern and Southern California. In this HMO membership, virtually all (96%) of the women used OC formula-tions containing <50 μg of ethinyl estradiol. Researchers identified all fatal and nonfatal strokes that occurred between 1991 and 1994 among female members between the ages of 15 and 44 years. Controls came from the same population.

A total of 408 confirmed strokes occurred among 1.1 million women during 3.6 million woman-years of observation. Of the

Figure 11

Adjusted Odds Ratios for Ischemic, Hemorrhagic, and All Types of Stroke According to Use of Oral Contraceptives in the Kaiser Permanente Population

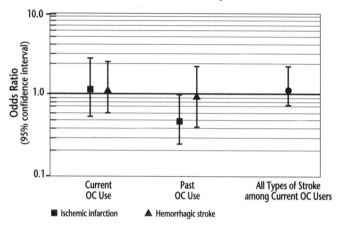

Source: Petitti DB, et al, 1996 (see reference 1).

identified stroke patients, interviews were completed for 357. Those with venous strokes or strokes of unknown type were excluded from final analyses in order to focus on arterial vascular disease. Women who had had hysterectomies or were pregnant at the time of the stroke were dropped from analysis. Multivariate analyses adjusted for major independent risk factors for stroke: cigarette smoking, hypertension, and diabetes.

The study found no increase in the overall risk of arterial stroke (either ischemic or hemorrhagic) among current low-dose OC users (Figure 11). On the basis of data from 295 women with stroke and their controls, the adjusted odds ratio (OR) for ischemic stroke among current users (as compared to former users and those who had never used OCs) was 1.2 (95% CI, 0.5-2.6). The adjusted odds ratio for hemorrhagic stroke was 1.1 (95% CI, 0.6-2.2). Past users had no increased risk of stroke. In fact, past users had a signifi-cantly *decreased* risk of ischemic stroke compared to never users (OR=0.5; 95% CI, 0.3-0.98)

Findings were similar for the subgroup of women who had subarachnoid hemorrhage. Among current users compared with former and never users, the odds ratio was 1.5 (95% CI, 0.6-3.6).

Three studies published since 1992 also compared current OC users with former and never users for the risk of having a subarachnoid hemorrhage. In those studies, the adjusted relative risk among current OC users was 1.1 (95% CI, 0.6-1.9) in the Thorogood and Mann study; the odds ratio was 0.9 (95% CI, 0.2-3.6) in Longstreth; and in the Royal College of General Practitioners' (RCGP) study, the largest and longest term of the three, the odds ratio was 1.5 (95% CI, 0.6-3.7).[4-6]

Smoking or Hypertension

The Kaiser Permanente study found a positive interaction between current OC use and smoking with respect to hemorrhagic stroke (p=0.04), but not ischemic stroke. Petitti et al reported an odds ratio for hemorrhagic stroke of 3.6 (95% CI, 0.95-13.9) among OC users who smoked as compared to a ratio of 0.8 (95% CI, 0.4-1.7) among those who did not smoke.

What about the link between stroke, OC use, and hypertension? In the Kaiser sample, so few current OC users also had hypertension that the researchers were unable to estimate a combined odds ratio for that subgroup.

WHO Data from Europe and Developing Countries

Data from Europe and developing countries are also reassuring that low-dose OCs do not cause stroke among healthy women.[2,3] The WHO Collaborative Study of Cardiovascular Disease and Steroid Hormone Contraception assessed the risk of MI and VTE, in addition to the risk of stroke. Overall, the study population comprised 3,792 identified cases of stroke, MI, and VTE, and 10,281 age-matched, hospitalized controls.

This hospital-based study assessed the odds ratios for ischemic stroke based on 697 identified cases, and for hemorrhagic stroke based on 1,068 identified cases. The study took place over a 4-year period, completed in June of 1993, across 17 countries in Europe, Africa, Asia, and Latin America. The latter three regions comprised developing countries.

One of the unique features of the WHO study was its high proportion of cases with accurate diagnosis of stroke. The diagnosis of ischemic stroke, for example, rested almost exclusively (97% to 100%) upon computed tomography, magnetic resonance imaging, or cerebral angiography carried out within 3 weeks of the clinical event. The diagnosis of hemorrhagic stroke by these methods ranged between 85% and 90%, except in Africa, where only 24% of cases could be diagnosed in this manner. Approximately 30% of the strokes studied were ischemic; 20% were unclassified, primarily among the African population, whose diagnostic facilities were inadequate; and the remainder were hemorrhagic.

Estrogen Dose

Any type of stroke

Were low-dose pills associated with a lower risk of stroke than high-dose pills? The WHO investigation found such a pattern in European users, but not in their counterparts in developing countries. In Europe, the odds ratio for any type of stroke associated with current use of low-dose OCs was elevated, but nonsignificant (OR=1.4; 95% CI, 0.9-2.2); in contrast, the risk associated with higher-dose OC use was significant, at 2.7 (95% CI, 1.7-4.3).

Ischemic and hemorrhagic stroke

European users of low-dose pills had no significantly increased risk of either ischemic or hemorrhagic stroke (Figure 12). Among European women, users of high-dose pills had a significantly increased risk of ischemic stroke (OR=5.3; 95% CI, 2.6-11).

Smoking

Cigarette smoking alone has been shown to increase the risk of stroke.[7] Furthermore, the risk of cardiovascular events has been shown to increase with smoking among OC users, particularly those over age 35 years.[8] The WHO investigation supports this finding. Nonsmoking European low-dose pill users were at no significantly increased risk of hemorrhagic stroke (OR=1.1, 95% CI, 0.5-2.5).

Odds ratios for ischemic stroke were highest among women who smoked. In Europe, OC users who smoked had over three times the risk of ischemic stroke (OR=7.2; 95% CI, 3.2-16.1) as OC

Figure 12

Adjusted Odds Ratios for Ischemic and Hemorrhagic Stroke in European Users of Oral Contraceptives by Estrogen Dose

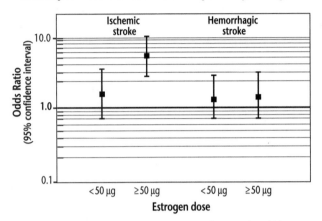

Source: World Health Organization, 1996 (see references 2 and 3).

users who did not smoke (OR=2.1; 95% CI, 1.0-4.5). Similarly, in developing countries, the odds ratio for ischemic stroke was about twice as high for smoking (OR=4.8; 95% CI, 2.8-8.4) as compared to nonsmoking OC users (OR=2.6; 95% CI, 1.9-3.8).

Hypertension

As with smoking, hypertension is an independent risk factor for stroke.[9] The WHO investigation found significantly increased risks of stroke, both ischemic and hemorrhagic, among women who had a history of hypertension. This was true of both OC users and nonusers. The risk of ischemic stroke was about four times higher, however, among European OC users who also had a history of hypertension (OR=10.7; 95% CI, 2.0-56.6), compared to OC users who had no history of hypertension (OR=2.7; 95% CI, 1.5-5.0).

Attributable Risk vs Relative Risk

The importance of attributable risk versus relative risk is critical when looking at an outcome measure that is rare (such as stroke in young women). Relative risks (and odds ratios) can be misleading without consideration of disease frequency.[10] For example, a relative risk of 3.0, indicating a tripling of risk, may sound alarming. When applied to a disease with an incidence of one per 100,000 women, however, that translates into an attributable risk of two cases per 100,000 women. In contrast, a small relative risk applied to a common disease may have the opposite effect. A relative risk of 1.2 (barely elevated) applied to a disease with a frequency of 1,000 per 100,000 women would yield an attributable risk of 200 cases per 100,000 women. In this latter example, the smaller relative risk would cause much more disease.

Take Home Messages

- *Both the US and international findings support the safety of low-dose OCs with regard to stroke, especially among healthy, nonsmoking women*

- *Like their US counterparts, nonsmoking European women using low-dose OCs did not have a significantly increased risk of either ischemic or hemorrhagic stroke*

- *Independent risk factors, such as smoking and hypertension, markedly increased the risk of stroke among OC users and nonusers*

- *The absolute risk of stroke among all women of reproductive age is very low, so even if a slightly increased risk exists with OC use, the attributable risk is very small*

References

1. Petitti DB, Sidney S, Bernstein A, et al. Stroke in users of low-dose oral contraceptives. *N Engl J Med* 1996;335:8-15.

2. WHO Collaborative Study of Cardiovascular Disease and Steroid Hormone Contraception. Ischaemic stroke and combined oral contraceptives: results of an international, multicentre, case-control study. *Lancet* 1996;348:498-505.

3. WHO Collaborative Study of Cardiovascular Disease and Steroid Hormone Contraception. Haemorrhagic stroke, overall stroke risk, and combined oral contraceptives: results of an international, multicentre, case-control study. *Lancet* 1996;348:505-510.

4. Thorogood M, Mann J, Murphy M, et al. Fatal stroke and use of oral contraceptives: findings from a case-control study. *Am J Epidemiol* 1992;136:35-45.

5. Longstreth WT, Nelson LM, Koepsell TD, et al. Subarachnoid hemorrhage and hormonal factors in women: a population-based case-control study. *Ann Intern Med* 1994;121:168-173.

6.   Hannaford PC, Croft PR, Kay CR. Oral contraception and stroke: evidence from the Royal College of General Practitioners' Oral Contraception Study. *Stroke* 1994;25:935-942.

7.   Shinton R, Beevers G. Meta-analysis of relation between cigarette smoking and stroke. *BMJ* 1989;298:789-794.

8.   Goldbaum GM, Kendrick JS, Hogelin GC, et al. The relative impact of smoking and oral contraceptive use on women in the United States. *JAMA* 1987;258:1339-1342.

9.   MacMahon S, Peto R, Cutler J, et al. Blood pressure, stroke, and coronary heart disease. Part I. Prolonged differences in blood pressure: prospective observational studies corrected for the regression dilution bias. *Lancet* 1990; 335:765-774.

10. Nakayama T, Zaman MM, Tanaka H. Reporting of attributable and relative risks, 1966-1997. *Lancet* 1998;351:1179. Letter.

iii. Myocardial Infarction

New data reconfirm the safety of oral contraceptives with regard to myocardial infarction. Nonsmoking women who are free of cardiovascular risk factors and have their blood pressure monitored before and during OC use have no increased risk of MI. Data also confirm that past use of OCs does not result in higher overall mortality or later cardiovascular disease of any type.

Past Use

Past use of OCs, even many years of use, does not increase a woman's overall mortality risk. The Nurses' Health Study, a large, prospective cohort study of 121,700 women who were ages 30 to 55 years in 1976, followed participants through 1988 (1.3 million person-years of follow-up).[1] No difference in overall mortality was found among women who had ever used OCs as compared with women who never had. When adjusted for age, body mass index, and cigarette smoking, the overall mortality relative risk (RR) was 0.9 (95% CI, 0.9-1.0). Long durations of OC use also conferred no risk. Women who had used OCs for 10 or more years had a relative risk of 1.1 (95% CI, 0.8-1.4).

Furthermore, a multivariate analysis found no increased risk for coronary heart disease, other heart disease, or stroke (Figure 13). This confirmed previous findings from the Nurses' Health Study and a meta-analysis of 13 additional studies that past use of OCs,

Figure 13

Cardiovascular Mortality and Past Use of Oral Contraceptives

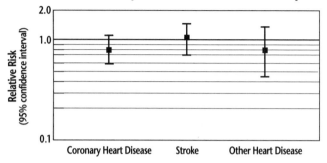

Source: Colditz GA, 1994 (see reference 1).

even for long periods, does not result in an increased risk of cardiovascular disease.[2,3]

Current Use and Cardiovascular Mortality

A recent Family Health International analysis estimated the risk of death from cardiovascular disease that can be attributed to low-dose OCs.[4] The researchers modeled estimates from studies published in the medical literature through 1997 and from age-specific mortality rates in the US for 1993 and 1994. The results indicate virtually no excess attributable risk of death from cardiovascular disease related to OC use in young women (<35 years). Women age 35 years or older who use OCs and smoke cigarettes, however, have a higher mortality rate from cardiovascular disease than women carrying a pregnancy to term.

Recent Evidence from the United States and Europe

Data from a large US health plan are reassuring with regard to the overall risk of MI among low-dose OC users. Sidney et al performed a population-based, case-control study of women aged 15 to 44 years enrolled in the California Kaiser Permanente Medical Care Program (Northern and Southern regions).[5] Cases were obtained during a 39-month period from 1991 through 1994. Members of the Kaiser plan are from ethnic backgrounds that

Figure 14

Estimated Incidence of First-Ever Myocardial Infarction in Women Aged 15 to 44 Years from the Kaiser Permanente Medical Care Program*—1991-1994

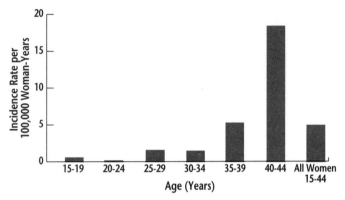

*Southern and Northern California regions

Source: Petitti DB, et al, 1997 (see reference 6).

generally represent the entire population of California. About 54% are white, non-Hispanic; 20%, Hispanic; 12%, African-American; 10%, Asian; and 4%, other and unknown.

The incidence of MI (excluding those occurring during pregnancy) was five per 100,000 woman-years (187 cases during 3.6 million woman-years of observation).[6] Myocardial infarction was very rare until age 35 years and only increased substantially among women aged 40 to 44 years (Figure 14). The researchers estimate that the attributable risk of MI among women aged 15 to 44 years from low-dose OC use is less than three cases per 1 million woman-years. This means that if 1 million women of reproductive age used OCs for 1 year, three women would die from an MI during that year who otherwise would not have died.

The odds ratio for MI in current OC users compared with non-current users was 1.7 (95% CI, 0.45-6.1).[5] (Noncurrent users were defined as women not currently using OCs, but who may have used them in the past.) For current use compared to no use, the OR was 1.1 (95% CI, 0.3-4.7) (Figure 15). Past use also was not associated

Figure 15

Adjusted Odds Ratios for Myocardial Infarction According to Oral Contraceptive Use, Kaiser Permanente Medical Care Program*—1991-1994

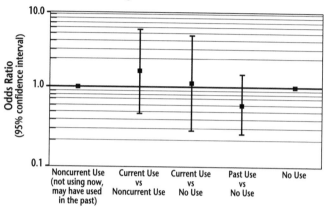

*Southern and Northern California regions

Source: Sidney S, et al, 1996 (see reference 5).

with any increased risk of MI. The wide confidence intervals reflect the overall rarity of MI in reproductive age women. A subsequent review of all MI studies by Petitti et al also concluded that past OC use does not increase the risk of MI.[7]

A large, case-control investigation by WHO found no significant risk of MI among OC users who did not smoke and also had their blood pressure checked before beginning OC use.[8] WHO also found no consistent pattern of increasing risk of myocardial infarction in OC users with advancing age or with increasing doses of estrogen.

Cigarette Smoking

Cigarette smoking greatly increases the likelihood of having an MI. Several investigations have found an interaction between smoking, OC use, and an increased risk of myocardial infarction. Rosenberg et al, for example, performed a case-control analysis of 555 women under the age of 50 years who survived their first MI.[9]

Figure 16

Estimated Relative Risk of Myocardial Infarction in Current OC Users According to Smoking Status — Royal College of General Practitioners' Oral Contraception Study

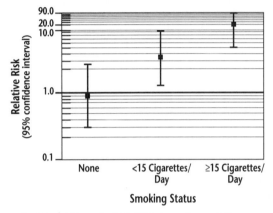

Source: Croft P and Hannaford PC, 1989 (see reference 10).

Nonsmoking OC users had no increased risk of MI; however, smoking substantially increased the risk of MI in general and among women using OCs. Light smokers (<25 cigarettes/day) using OCs had three times the risk of MI, while heavy smokers (≥25 cigarettes/day) using OCs had 23 times the risk of nonsmoking OC users.

A reanalysis of the Royal College of General Practitioners' Oral Contraception Study also found no elevated risk of MI in current OC users who did not smoke.[10] Women who did not smoke and used OCs had an RR of 0.9 (95% CI, 0.3-2.7). Light smokers (<15 cigarettes/day) using OCs tripled their risk of MI and heavy smokers (≥15 cigarettes/day) using OCs had 20 times the risk as nonsmokers (Figure 16).

An analysis of MI and smoking found that most excess cases of myocardial infarction among US women aged 35 to 44 years can be attributed solely to smoking.[11] Furthermore, pregnancy carried to term is more dangerous than combined smoking and OC use, except for women aged 35 years and older.[4,11]

Myocardial infarction among OC users is clearly linked to cigarette smoking. The WHO analysis found that more than twice as many cases smoked cigarettes as did controls (77% vs 35%).[8] Compared with nonsmoking women who did not use OCs, OC users who smoked 10 or more cigarettes daily significantly and exponentially increased their risk of MI in Europe (OR=87; 95% CI, 30-254) and in developing countries (OR=23; 95% CI, 8-67).

Patients should be encouraged to stop smoking rather than discontinue OCs. Women under the age of 35 years who smoke may use OCs, but should be warned about the dangers of smoking. Women 35 years of age or older who smoke and cannot quit should be encouraged to use another method of birth control. Counseling from clinicians, nicotine replacement therapies, and the antidepressant bupropion can help patients quit smoking.

Progestin Type

One study has also suggested that the risk of MI differs between levonorgestrel-containing pills and those containing the progestins desogestrel and gestodene. The Transnational Research Group Study on Oral Contraceptives and the Health of Young Women published its final results in 1997.[12] The study found a statistically significant difference between the occurrence of MI in users of "third-" vs "second-generation" pills (OR= 0.3; 95% CI, 0.1-0.9). Third-generation OCs were defined as those containing desogestrel and gestodene; second-generation OCs were defined as those containing all other progestins. A separate analysis also compared levonorgestrel-containing OCs with third-generation OCs.

A heated debate followed.[13-17] The finding was based on a small number of women with MI (n=7) taking the new progestin pills. Arguments suggested that OCs containing gestodene and desogestrel were just as safe as levonorgestrel products because the potential increased risk of VTE was offset by the reduced risk of MI.[13,14] Furthermore, some suggested that the morbidity and mortality from VTE was less than that from MI and, thus, the MI data should be given greater weight when evaluating the risk-to-benefit ratio. (For further discussion, see the section on venous thromboembolism.)

Three facts limit conclusions that can be drawn from the Transnational results, however. First, only seven cases were third-generation pill users. Second, 80% of the cases were smokers, while only about 35% of controls smoked. Because of the small number of MI cases, the data could not be stratified for cigarette smoking within each progestin category, limiting the interpretation of the results. Third, the difference only held up when community controls were used as the comparison group. When hospital controls were used, on the other hand, the relative risks for MI were almost identical for third- and second-generation pills and for levonorgestrel-containing OCs.

Follow-up data also are unable to confirm a statistically significant effect of type of progestin on MI risk. These data come from the WHO investigation in Europe and developing countries,[8] from the United States,[5] and from an analysis of the United Kingdom (UK) General Practitioners' Database.[18] Furthermore, animal experiments suggest that a levonorgestrel-containing triphasic OC may help to protect against arterial thrombotic events, such as MI and stroke.[19]

Because of the controversy, WHO recently reviewed the evidence concerning cardiovascular events and OCs.[20] WHO noted the general safety of OCs, especially when used in nonsmoking women without other cardiovascular risk factors who have their blood pressure checked. With regard to MI, WHO stated that in such women, the risk of MI in users of combined OCs is not increased, regardless of age. WHO also found the available data do not allow a conclusion that the risk of MI in users of low-dose combined OCs is related to progestin type.

Take Home Messages

- OCs do not increase the risk of myocardial infarction in non-smoking, normotensive women
- Cigarette smoking is the greatest risk factor for myocardial infarction among reproductive age women
- All women should be encouraged to stop smoking rather than stop using OCs
- Women 35 years of age or older who cannot stop smoking should be encouraged to use another method of birth control

Continued on next page

Take Home Messages (continued)

- *Clinician recommendation to stop smoking is very important and should be repeated at each visit*

- *Women should be screened for high blood pressure before prescribing OCs, with options evaluated for hypertensive individuals*

- *The available data on risk of MI do not demonstrate any definitive benefit or risk based on type of progestin; no change in prescribing habits or clinical practice is warranted*

References

1. Colditz GA and The Nurses' Health Study Research Group. Oral contraceptive use and mortality during 12 years of follow-up: the Nurses' Health Study. *Ann Intern Med* 1994;120:821-826.

2. Stampfer MJ, Willett WC, Colditz GA, et al. A prospective study of past use of oral contraceptive agents and risk of cardiovascular diseases. *N Engl J Med* 1988;319:1313-1317.

3. Stampfer MJ, Willett WC, Colditz GA, et al. Past use of oral contraceptives and cardiovascular disease: a meta-analysis in the context of the Nurses' Health Study. *Am J Obstet Gynecol* 1990;163:285-291.

4. Schwingl PJ, Ory HW, Visness CM. Estimates of the risk of cardiovascular death attributable to low-dose oral contraceptives in the United States. *Am J Obstet Gynecol* 1999;180:241-249.

5. Sidney S, Petitti DB, Quesenberry CP Jr., et al. Myocardial infarction in users of low-dose oral contraceptives. *Obstet Gynecol* 1996;88:939-944.

6. Petitti DB, Sidney S, Quesenberry CP Jr., et al. Incidence of stroke and myocardial infarction in women of reproductive age. *Stroke* 1997;28:280-283.

7. Petitti DB, Sidney S, Quesenberry CP Jr. Oral contraceptive use and myocardial infarction. *Contraception* 1998;57:143-155.

8. WHO Collaborative Study of Cardiovascular Disease and Steroid Hormone Contraception. Acute myocardial infarction and combined oral contraceptives: results of an international muticentre case-control study. *Lancet* 1997; 349:1202-1209.

9. Rosenberg L, Kaufman DW, Helmrich SP, et al. Myocardial infarction and cigarette smoking in women younger than 50 years of age. *JAMA* 1985;253: 2965-2969.

10. Croft P, Hannaford PC. Risk factors for acute myocardial infarction in women: evidence from the Royal College of General Practitioners' Oral Contraceptive Study. *BMJ* 1989;298:165-168.

11. Goldbaum GM, Kendrick JS, Hogelin GC, et al. The relative impact of smoking and oral contraceptive use on women in the United States. *JAMA* 1987;258:1339-1342.

12. Lewis MA, Heinemann LAJ, Spitzer WO, et al. The use of oral contraceptives and the occurrence of acute myocardial infarction in young women. *Contraception* 1997;56:129-140.

13. Lewis MA, Spitzer WO, Heinemann LAJ, et al. Lowered risk of dying of heart attack with third generation pill may offset risk of dying of thromboembolism. *BMJ* 1997;315:679-680.

14. Schwingl PJ, Shelton J. Modeled estimates of myocardial infarction and venous thromboembolic disease in users of second and third generation oral contraceptives. *Contraception* 1997;55:125-129.

15. Lewis MAF, Heinemann LAJ, MacRae KD, et al. The increased risk of venous thromboembolism and the use of third generation progestagens: role of bias in observational research. *Contraception* 1996;54:5-13.

16. Suissa S, Blais L, Spitzer WO, et al. First-time use of newer oral contraceptives and the risk of venous thromboembolism. *Contraception* 1997;56: 141-146.

17. Farley TMM, Meirik O, Marmot MG, et al. Oral contraceptives and risk of venous thromboembolism: impact of duration of use. *Contraception* 1998; 57:61-64. Letter.

18. Jick H, Jick SS, Myers MW. Risk of acute myocardial infarction and low-dose combined oral contraceptives. *Lancet* 1996;347:627-628.

19. Bellinger DA, Williams JK, Adams MR, et al. Oral contraceptives and hormone replacement therapy do not increase the incidence of arterial thrombosis in a nonhuman primate model. *Arterioscler Thromb Vasc Biol* 1998;18:92-99.

20. World Health Organization. WHO Scientific Group meeting on cardiovascular disease and steroid hormone contraceptives. *Wkly Epidemiol Rec* 1997; No.48:361-363.

iv. Venous Thromboembolism

Oral contraceptives containing desogestrel and gestodene may carry a small risk of venous thromboembolism that exceeds the risk associated with OCs containing older progestins. If true, this risk is still only half of the VTE risk associated with pregnancy—one of the key reasons why neither the US Food and Drug Administration nor the American College of Obstetricians and Gynecologists (ACOG) recommends switching current users of desogestrel-containing OCs to other products. (OCs containing gestodene are not currently available in the US.)

In October 1995, the prescription drug regulatory agency in the UK, the Committee on Safety of Medicines, issued a warning to health care providers and patients. Data leaked to the media from several large, then-unpublished studies had suggested that combination oral contraceptives containing the newer progestins desogestrel or gestodene were associated with about twice the risk of VTE compared with OCs containing older progestins, such as levonorgestrel.[1-5] (No relative risk was initially reported for the progestin norgestimate because of its rare use in Europe.) The move touched off great concern among practitioners and patients. In Europe, OC use dropped and the number of induced abortions rose. A heated debate ensued as to whether study bias contributed to the VTE risk findings.[6-11]

Disagreement over the findings still lingers. While some believe the link is based on firm evidence, others dismiss the concerns, citing probable biases. A recent comprehensive review that emerged from a WHO Scientific Group meeting examined the original studies, their main findings, the arguments in favor of bias, and reanalyses and counterarguments. That review, however, asserts that biases cannot account for the results entirely (Table 14).[12]

Several biases have been offered as explanations for the increased risk of VTE found in the studies of desogestrel- and gestodene-containing OCs. The types of bias offered as explanations include attrition of susceptibles (the healthy user effect or recency of introduction bias), selective prescribing (selection bias), and preferential diagnosis, among others.

For example, selection or prescribing bias may have occurred if clinicians steered women at higher risk of thromboembolic complications, such as obese women, toward the newer pills, believing newer pills to be safer. Researchers note, however, that few clinical risk factors predict the likelihood of venous thrombosis in healthy young women. This makes it less likely that clinicians could have identified high-risk patients and targeted them for prescriptions of newer OCs.[13] One obvious risk factor is previous VTE, but the studies in question were limited to first thrombosis. Those risk factors believed to be the strongest predictors of first VTE—positive family history, gross obesity, and factor V Leiden mutation—were either accounted for in the studies or, as in the case of factor V Leiden, were all but unknown at the time of patient entry (Table 15).[13] Adjusting for these risk factors had little effect on the results of the studies.

Another type of bias is attrition of susceptibles or the healthy user effect. This type of bias may have occurred because women taking levonorgestrel-containing pills were longer-term users.

Table 14

VTE Studies: Findings, Potential Biases, and Responses

Study	Main Finding	Potential Bias	Response
WHO Collaborative[1]	Current OC use was associated with a three- to fourfold increased risk of VTE.	Results could have been confounded by age differences between cases and controls.	The authors reanalyzed their data with more exact age matching. Findings did not differ substantially from the original report.
UK General Practice Research Database[3]	In the nested case-control analysis, the adjusted matched relative risk estimates were twice as high for desogestrel and gestodene users compared with levonorgestrel users.	Study was based on information in a computerized database. These data tend to be incomplete and not as meticulously gathered as in a clinical trial.	The database was used primarily to identify patients. Treating physicians were then contacted directly for further case details, such as hospitalizations and specialist referrals.
Leiden Thrombophilia[4]	OCs containing desogestrel were associated with about a ninefold increased risk of VTE compared with nonusers (2.3 times greater risk than levonorgestrel).	Risk factors such as family history of deep vein thrombosis (DVT) can result in preferential prescribing of newer pill formulations (selection bias).	Risk ratios for desogestrel-containing OCs were similar among women with and without a family history of DVT, as well as other risk factors.
Transnational[5]	Third-generation OCs were associated with nearly a fivefold increased risk of VTE compared with nonusers (1.5 times greater risk than second-generation OCs).	Some argued that the study failed to account for shorter average durations of use for OCs with newer progestins, which resulted in an artificially inflated risk.	Methodological refinements did not lead to a different conclusion.

Source: Walker AM, 1998 (see reference 12).

Table 15

VTE Risk Factors

- Prior venous thromboembolic events
- Clotting abnormalities, such as factor V Leiden
- Obesity
- Positive family history
- Immobilization
- Recent surgery
- Cancer
- Chronic medical conditions

Long-term users, as a group, tend to include fewer women likely to experience problems with the pill, as those women who have side effects discontinue OC use early. Younger, first-time users are, thus, at greater risk of experiencing VTE. Some evidence suggests that young, first-time users were more likely to have taken the newer pills. Furthermore, one analysis also found that the risk of VTE for different OC formulations increased linearly and significantly with recency of market introduction.[9]

Critics have countered that the findings supporting attrition of susceptibles in the Transnational data only applied to one age category.[12,13] Higher risk with more recently introduced products was limited to women aged 25 to 44 years, about half of the subjects studied.[9] This trend is not seen in the overall data set. Moreover, data for subjects under the age of 25 years revealed a trend opposite of that observed in the group of older women, weakening the argument further.[12]

Other Objections

Biological plausibility

Researchers have also argued that no plausible biological explanation exists for finding higher VTE risk with OCs containing newer progestins.[6] Indeed, given that progestins are not thrombogenic, how particular progestins could increase the risk of VTE is unclear.

In response, other researchers have made two assertions. First, some note that the lack of *in vitro* support for a hypothesis that is based on real-world observation is not a critical flaw, nor is it without precedent in drug research.[12] Second, others have suggested that the less "androgenic" (or, more accurately, less "antiestrogenic") effect of newer progestins may actually result in a more "estrogenic" pill, which could account for the increased relative risk for VTE.

The 20 μg paradox

In several of the original studies, the greatest risk was found among new OC formulations containing 20 μg, rather than 30 μg, of ethinyl estradiol. This was also true in a more recent analysis using a proprietary database known as MediPlus.[14] Given that it is illogical to find the highest VTE risk with the lowest estrogen dose (vs formulations containing the same progestins and 30 μg EE), researchers have argued this reflects bias, not biology.

Drawing Conclusions

As long as questions remain unanswered and a plausible biological explanation continues to elude researchers, the issue may never be fully resolved.

The FDA has adopted the position that the potential added VTE risk is not great enough to justify switching to other products.[15] ACOG took a similar stance in December 1996; the group did not recommend that women change their brand of OC.[16] A 1998 ACOG amended review further states that OCs containing desogestrel are acceptable for new starts.[17]

In April 1999, the UK's Committee on Safety of Medicines and Medicines Control Agency revised statements concerning the risk of VTE associated with OCs containing desogestrel or gestodene.[18] The agency said it "regretted" the increase in abortions that followed the pill scare of 1995. The agency revised product information to state, "The absolute risk of VTE in women taking combination OCs containing desogestrel or gestodene is very small and is much less than the risk of VTE in pregnancy. Provided that women are fully informed of these very small risks and do not have medical contraindications, it should be a matter of clinical judgment and personal choice which type of oral contraceptive should be prescribed."[19]

Placing Risk in Perspective

Despite the FDA's position, in 1996, manufacturers of desogestrel-containing products amended package labeling to include a

Figure 17

Estimated Average Risk of Nonfatal Venous Thromboembolism per 100,000 Women per Year, US

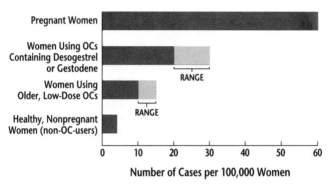

Source: US Food and Drug Administration, 1995 (see reference 15).

warning about a possible increased risk of VTE. If real, this increased risk needs perspective. According to the FDA, the estimated average risk of nonfatal VTE is four cases per 100,000 per year among women who do not use oral contraceptives (Figure 17). On the other hand, about 10 to 15 cases per 100,000 per year occur among users of older, low-dose OCs. Even if OCs containing newer progestins carry twice the VTE risk, the resulting nonfatal VTE incidence of 20 to 30 per 100,000 is still only half the estimated VTE risk for pregnant women (60 per 100,000).[15]

Counseling Suggestions

- *If patients are already using a desogestrel-containing OC and do not have risk factors for VTE, no change is necessary; clinicians may want to mention the issue to these patients, adding that the excess risk, if any, is small*

- *For new starts, take a personal and family history to help determine VTE risk; in the absence of risk factors, proceed as usual*

- *If a desogestrel-containing OC is prescribed, inform the patient of the possibility of increased risk of VTE*

Continued on next page

Counseling Suggestions (continued)

- Counsel all OC users to report signs and symptoms of VTE:
    - Shortness of breath
    - Difficulty breathing
    - Pain or swelling in the leg

- If patients have a personal history of VTE, they should not be prescribed combination OCs

- If patients have a strong positive family history of VTE (young first- and second-degree relatives) or exhibit other risk factors (eg, obesity, immobilization), clinicians should, depending upon the number and severity of the risk factors, consider a birth control method other than combined OCs

- Counsel patients about the health benefits of OCs to help give a balanced perspective

---

Take Home Messages

- Low-dose OC users have about a three- to fourfold increased risk of VTE compared to nonusers

- OCs containing desogestrel and gestodene may (or may not) carry a small risk of VTE that exceeds the risk associated with OCs containing older progestins

- Debate concerning the data continues, with arguments made both for and against bias

- The FDA and ACOG do not recommend changes in prescribing

References

1. WHO Collaborative Study of Cardiovascular Disease and Steroid Hormone Contraception. Venous thromboembolic disease and combined oral contraceptives: results of international multicentre case-control study. *Lancet* 1995;346:1575-1582.

2. WHO Collaborative Study of Cardiovascular Disease and Steroid Hormone Contraception. Effect of different progestagens in low oestrogen oral contraceptives on venous thromboembolic disease. *Lancet* 1995;346:1582-1588.

3. Jick H, Jick SS, Gurewich V, et al. Risk of idiopathic cardiovascular death and nonfatal venous thromboembolism in women using oral contraceptives with differing progestagen components. *Lancet* 1995;346:1589-1593.

4. Bloemenkamp KMW, Rosendaal FR, Helmerhorst FM, et al. Enhancement by factor V Leiden mutation of risk of deep vein thrombosis associated with oral contraceptives containing a third-generation progestagen. *Lancet* 1995; 346:1593-1596.

5. Spitzer WO, Lewis MA, Heinemann LAJ, et al. Third generation oral contraceptives and risk of venous thromboembolic disorders: an international case-control study. *BMJ* 1996;312:83-88.

6. Rosenberg L, Palmer JR, Sands MI, et al. Modern oral contraceptives and cardiovascular disease. *Am J Obstet Gynecol* 1997;177:707-715.

7. Heinemann LAJ, Lewis MA. Increased risk estimates for venous thromboembolism under oral contraceptives with third-generation progestagens due to preferential prescribing? *Pharmacoepidemiol Drug Safety* 1996;5:599.

8. Dunn N, White I, Freemantle S, et al. The role of prescribing and referral bias in studies of the association between third-generation oral contraceptives and increased risk of thromboembolism. *Pharmacoepidemiol Drug Safety* 1998;7:3-14.

9. Lewis MA, Heinemann LAJ, MacRae KD, et al. The increased risk of venous thromboembolism and the use of third-generation progestagens: role of bias in observational research. *Contraception* 1996;54:5-13.

10. Suissa S, Blais L, Spitzer WO, et al. First-time use of newer oral contraceptives and the risk of venous thromboembolism. *Contraception* 1997;56:141-146.

11. Bloemenkamp KW, Rosendaal FR, Buller HR, et al. Risk of venous thrombosis with use of current low-dose oral contraceptives is not explained by diagnostic suspicion and referral bias. *Arch Intern Med* 1998;159:65-70.

12. Walker AM. Newer oral contraceptives and the risk of venous thromboembolism. *Contraception* 1998;57:169-181.

13. Vandenbroucke JP, Helmerhorst FM, Bloemenkamp KMW, et al. Third-generation oral contraceptive and deep venous thrombosis: from epidemiologic controversy to new insight in coagulation. *Am J Obstet Gynecol* 1997;177: 887-891.

14. Farmer RDT, Lawrenson RA, Thompson CR, et al. Population-based study of risk of venous thromboembolism associated with various oral contraceptives. *Lancet* 1997;349:83-88.

15. Food and Drug Administration. Oral contraceptives and the risk of blood clots. *FDA Talk Paper* Nov. 24, 1995.

16. American College of Obstetricians and Gynecologists. Gyn committee assesses VTE and oral contraceptive link. *ACOG Newsletter* 1996;40:(12).

17. American College of Obstetricians and Gynecologists. ACOG committee revises recommendations on OCs with third-generation progestins. *ACOG Today* 1998;42:(6).

18. Rumbelow H. Government U-turn on pill warning. *The Times* (UK) April 8, 1999.

19. Committee on Safety of Medicines and the Medicines Control Agency. Combined oral contraceptives containing desogestrel or gestodene and the risk of venous thromboembolism. *Curr Prob Pharmacovigilance* 1999;25.

v. Venous Thromboembolism Screening

Much debate surrounds whether first-time pill users should be screened for genetic markers that might predispose them to thrombotic episodes. Most evidence indicates that such a policy is neither practical nor cost-effective. Instead, clinicians should take a personal and family history of venous thromboembolism prior to prescribing oral contraceptives.

Several inherited abnormalities of the hemostatic system increase the risk of VTE. These are present in approximately one-third of all cases of spontaneous VTE within the Caucasian population.[1] Given the slightly elevated risk of VTE among OC users, questions have been raised concerning screening women for thrombophilic mutations before prescribing OCs.[2-5]

Known Thrombophilic Markers

The most common known genetic cause of thrombophilia is the factor V Leiden mutation,[4,6] a defect first identified in 1993.[7,8] Factor V Leiden falls into the category of thrombophilic mutations also known as activated protein C (APC) resistance. Factor V Leiden thrombophilia is present in about one-quarter (23%) of Caucasian women with spontaneous VTE.

Other thrombophilic markers include deficiencies in anticoagulation proteins, such as protein C, protein S, and antithrombin III. Compared with factor V Leiden, however, these additional markers are rare; together, they are found in only about 8% of women experiencing a first episode of spontaneous VTE (Figure 18).[1]

Scale and Consequences of Screening

Substantial challenges limit the practicality and utility of widespread screening for thrombophilic mutations. First, more than two-thirds (70%) of all thromboembolic events are unrelated to any known genetic abnormality. As a result, screening prospective combination OC users for known thrombophilic markers would miss most women who would eventually develop a clot.

Second, factor V Leiden is present in fewer than 5% of asymptomatic US Caucasian women.[1] The prevalence in other races is considerably lower: Hispanic Americans, 2.2%; Native Americans,

Figure 18

Prevalence of Known Thrombophilic Markers among Caucasian Women Experiencing a First Episode of Spontaneous VTE

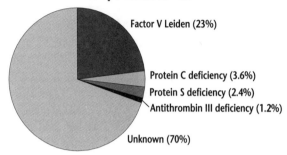

Factor V Leiden (23%)

Protein C deficiency (3.6%)
Protein S deficiency (2.4%)
Antithrombin III deficiency (1.2%)

Unknown (70%)

Source: Winkler UH, 1998 (see reference 1).

1.3%; African-Americans, 1.2%; and Asian Americans, 0.5%.[4,5] Consequently, a large number of women would have to be screened to identify a relatively small pool of factor V Leiden carriers. Furthermore, only a small number within this pool actually would develop combination OC-related thromboembolic events—resulting in a large number of "false positives." Knowledge of this thrombophilic marker also could stigmatize women, resulting in poorer perceived health and difficulty obtaining insurance.

One cost-effectiveness analysis by Creinin et al evaluated the proposed practice of screening US women using OCs for factor V Leiden.[9] The researchers estimated that over 92,000 carriers of this genetic thrombophilic marker would need to be identified and stopped from using OCs in order to prevent one death from VTE. The estimated cost of preventing this one death was estimated to be $300 million. The researchers concluded that the best available screening tool is a thorough personal and family history regarding venous thromboembolic events.

Other researchers have asserted that more than 2 million OC users would need to be screened to prevent a single OC-related VTE death, at a screening cost in excess of $100 million.[10] In the process, more than 120,000 women would be denied combined oral contraceptives and may have to resort to less effective methods of birth control. These women would, therefore, be at greater risk for pregnancy, which itself carries a greater risk of fatal VTE, potentially resulting in a "net medical hazard."[5,10]

VTE Personal and Family History Questions

- *Have you or a close family member (parents, siblings, grandparents, uncles, aunts) ever had blood clots in the legs or lungs?*

- *Have you or a close family member ever been hospitalized for blood clots in the legs or lungs?*

- *If so, did you or your family member take a blood thinner? (If not, the likelihood is that the family member may have had a nonsignificant condition, such as superficial phlebitis or varicose veins.)*

- *What were the circumstances in which the blood clot took place (eg, cancer, airline travel, obesity, immobility, recent pregnancy, etc)?*

Take Home Messages

- *Several inherited abnormalities of the hemostatic system, such as factor V Leiden, increase the risk of VTE*

- *Screening for thrombophilic markers before prescribing OCs, however, is neither practical nor cost-effective*

- *Clinicians should take a careful personal and family history of VTE before prescribing OCs*

- *If a patient has a VTE, testing for thrombophilic markers is indicated*

References

1. Winkler UH. Blood coagulation and oral contraceptives: a critical review. *Contraception* 1998;57:203-209.

2. Hellgren M, Svensson PJ, Dahlback B. Resistance to activated protein C as a basis for venous thromboembolism associated with pregnancy and oral contraceptives. *Am J Obstet Gynecol* 1995;173:210-213.

3. Schambeck CM, Schwender S, Haubitz I, et al. Selective screening for the factor V Leiden mutation: is it advisable prior to the prescription of oral contraceptives? *Thromb Haemost* 1997;78:1480-1483.

4. Vandenbroucke JP, van der Meer FJM, Helmerhorst FM, et al. Factor V Leiden: should we screen oral contraceptive users and pregnant women? *BMJ* 1996;313:1127-1130.

5. Price DT, Ridker PM. Factor V Leiden mutation and the risks for thromboembolic disease: a clinical perspective. *Ann Intern Med* 1997;127:895-903.

6. Zoller B, Dahlback B. Linkage between inherited resistance to activated protein C and factor V gene mutation in venous thrombosis. *Lancet* 1994; 343:1536-1538.

7. Dahlback B, Carlsson M, Svensson PJ. Familial thrombophilia due to a previously unrecognized mechanism characterized by poor anticoagulant response to activated protein C: prediction of a cofactor to activated protein C. *Proc Natl Acad Sci USA* 1993;90:1004-1008.

8. Koster T, Rosendaal FR, de Ronde H, et al. Venous thrombosis due to poor anticoagulant response to activated protein C: Leiden Thrombophilia Study. *Lancet* 1993;342:1503-1506.

9. Creinin MD, Lisman R, Strickler RC. Screening for factor V Leiden mutation before prescribing combination oral contraceptives. *Fertil Steril* 1999;72: 646-651.

10. Rosendaal FR. Oral contraceptives and screening for factor V Leiden. *Thromb Haemost* 1996;75:524-525.

2.3: Reproductive Cancers

i. Breast Cancer

Over the past 3 decades, numerous studies and reviews have attempted to quantify the relationship between oral contraceptives and breast cancer. Overall, the data have been reassuring, indicating no increased risk of breast cancer over a lifetime, whether the data were collected from cohort or case-control investigations.[1-8]

The largest-ever epidemiologic analysis provides strong evidence that OCs do not cause breast cancer. The Collaborative Group on Hormonal Factors in Breast Cancer gathered data on over 53,000 women with breast cancer and over 100,000 controls from 54 studies conducted in 26 countries. The researchers compiled their information from 90% of the known studies regarding the relationship between OCs and breast cancer. The findings were first published in *The Lancet*.[9] Detailed analyses then appeared in a supplement to the journal *Contraception*.[10] Two main findings emerged.

• Current users and those who have taken OCs within the past 10 years have a small increased risk of having breast cancer diagnosed (RR for current use=1.24; 99% CI, 1.20-1.28) (Figure 19).[10]

• Women have no significant excess risk of having breast cancer diagnosed 10 or more years after stopping use (RR at 10 years=1.0; 99% CI, 0.97-1.07).

After controlling for recency of use, the risk was essentially unchanged, despite numerous analyses for factors hypothesized to impact breast cancer risk. The following factors did not appreciably alter the risk of breast cancer:

• Duration of use	• Reproductive history
• Age at first use	• Family history of breast cancer
• Type of formulation	• Ethnic origin
• High vs low dose	• Height
• Parity	• Weight
• Age	• Menopausal status
• Age at menarche	• Alcohol use

Figure 19

Relative Risk of Breast Cancer Being Diagnosed in OC Users

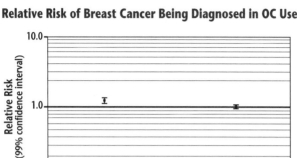

Source: *Collaborative Group on Hormonal Factors in Breast Cancer, 1996 (see reference 10).*

The lack of an association among duration of use, dose, and breast cancer risk supports the hypothesis that OCs do not cause the disease. Instead, the likelihood of diagnosis may be enhanced by closer surveillance of women who take OCs. Or, it may be that women taking OCs access health care services more frequently.

Women with a family history of breast cancer often fear using hormones. The findings indicate, however, that women with a family history of breast cancer (mother or sister) do not increase their risk of the disease by using OCs. Evidence also suggests that OCs do not increase the risk of developing breast cancer in women with benign breast disease.[7,8]

Importantly, the Collaborative Group also found that breast cancer tumors in OC users were more likely to be localized to the breast. Tumors were less likely to have spread beyond the breast among current OC users compared to never users (RR=0.85; 99% CI, 0.78-0.92).[9]

Diagnosing more localized tumors tends to support the hypothesis that OC users are screened more frequently and their tumors caught earlier than nonusers. An earlier diagnosis enhances successful treatment and long-term survival.

Take Home Messages

- *Evidence from the largest-ever epidemiologic analysis suggests that OCs do not cause breast cancer*

- *OC users and those who have stopped within the past 10 years are at a slightly increased risk of being diagnosed with breast cancer*

- *OC users in whom breast cancer is diagnosed have a greater likelihood of their tumors being localized than nonusers*

- *10 or more years after stopping use, an OC user's risk of breast cancer is the same as in a woman who has never used OCs*

- *OCs can be used by women with a family history of breast cancer or current benign breast disease*

- *Women often fear breast cancer and need reassurance about the latest evidence*

References

1. Committee on the Relationship between Oral Contraceptives and Breast Cancer. *Oral Contraceptives and Breast Cancer*. Institute of Medicine, Division of Health Promotion and Disease Prevention. Washington, DC: National Academy Press; 1991.

2. Thomas DB. Oral contraceptives and breast cancer: review of the epidemiological literature. In: *Oral Contraceptives and Breast Cancer*. Institute of Medicine, Division of Health Promotion and Disease Prevention. Washington, DC: National Academy Press; 1991.

3. Cancer and Steroid Hormone Study of the Centers for Disease Control and the National Institute of Child Health and Human Development. Oral contraceptive use and the risk of breast cancer. *N Engl J Med* 1986;315:405-411.

4. Royal College of General Practitioners. Breast cancer and oral contraceptives: findings in Royal College of General Practitioners' study. *BMJ* 1981;282:2089-2093.

5. Romieu I, Willett WC, Colditz GA, et al. Prospective study of oral contraceptive use and risk of breast cancer in women. *J Natl Cancer Inst* 1989;81:1313-1321.

6. WHO Collaborative Study of Neoplasia and Steroid Contraceptives. Breast cancer and combined oral contraceptives: results from a multi-national study. *Br J Cancer* 1990;61:110-119.

7. Schlesselman JJ. Oral contraceptives and breast cancer. *Am J Obstet Gynecol* 1990;163(pt 1):1379-1387.

8. Murray PP, Stadel BV, Schlesselman JJ. Oral contraceptive use in women with a family history of breast cancer. *Obstet Gynecol* 1989;73:977-983.

9. Collaborative Group on Hormonal Factors in Breast Cancer. Breast cancer and hormonal contraceptives: collaborative reanalysis of individual data on 53,297 women with breast cancer and 100,239 women without breast cancer from 54 epidemiological studies. *Lancet* 1996;347:1713-1727.

10. Collaborative Group on Hormonal Factors in Breast Cancer. Breast cancer and hormonal contraceptives: further results. *Contraception* 1996;54:1S-106S.

ii. Cervical Cancer

The exact relationship between oral contraceptive use and cervical cancer is not known, largely due to the complex etiology of this disease. It appears that long-term use of OCs (>5 years) may be associated with an increased risk of invasive disease; however, cervical cancer has been linked to factors other than OC use, including human papillomavirus (HPV), cigarette smoking, sexual behavior, lower socioeconomic status, and parity. Furthermore, biases and confounding variables have often been present in studies of cervical cancer in relation to OC use.[1]

Research on OCs and cervical cancer is subject to a variety of possible biases and confounding factors. Some of the major potential confounding variables that have influenced study results include sexual history, cigarette smoking, and HPV infection.

Sexual History

Strong evidence supports the hypothesis that cervical cancer is associated with one or more sexually transmitted diseases.[2] Intercourse at an early age, multiple sexual partners, and sexual behavior of partners also have been associated with cervical cancer development.[2,3]

Human Papillomavirus

Strong evidence suggests that certain strains of HPV cause cervical cancer. One study of 500 women with cervical intraepithelial neoplasia and 500 disease-free women attributed about 76% of cases to HPV infection.[4] Another case-control study from the Division for Cancer Epidemiology in Denmark estimated that 66% of cervical cancer cases could be attributed to HPV; however, when results were restricted to histologically confirmed high-grade lesions, the proportion increased to 80%.[5]

Parity

The likelihood of developing invasive cervical cancer has been shown in some studies to increase with number of births. In one study, the risk was found to double after just one birth; women with five or more births were four times more likely to develop cervical cancer than were nulliparous women.[6]

Smoking History

A large body of research exists regarding the possible effect of smoking on the development of cervical cancer. In a 1990 review of the literature, Winkelstein reported that almost 80% of the 33 cited studies supported an association.[7]

Pap Smear Frequency

In studies of the effect of OC use on cervical dysplasia and carcinoma *in situ*, frequency of Pap smears can be a source of bias that inflates relative risk estimates. OC users may receive Pap smears more regularly than nonusers. Thus, OC users may more likely be diagnosed with these two conditions than nonusers, resulting in a spuriously elevated relative risk.[1]

Disease Stage and Duration of Use

Collective data regarding both cervical dysplasia and carcinoma *in situ* are difficult to interpret, and evidence of an association between OCs and these two disease stages is weak.[8] Studies focusing on invasive cervical cancer and OCs have yielded conflicting results, although two reports from WHO, published in 1993 and 1996, suggest an association.[9-16]

The risk of invasive cervical cancer does not appear to be elevated during the first 5 years of oral contraceptive use.[9] An association is more likely to exist with durations of use greater than 5 years, with about a twofold increased risk at 10 years. Follow-up data from the Oxford Family Planning Association also suggest a significantly increased risk of all types of cervical neoplasia with 97 or more months of OC use (RR=2.0; 95% CI, 1.3-3.1).[17] Data from a population-based, case-control study from the Los Angeles (California) County Cancer Surveillance Program found similar results.[18]

The frequency of Pap smear screening continues to be debated. The American College of Obstetricians and Gynecologists and the American Cancer Society recommend annual screening. On the other hand, the US Preventive Services Task Force recommends screening at least once every 3 years, with the interval determined by the clinician based on the woman's risk factors for cervical cancer.

Take Home Messages

- Results of existing studies are inconclusive with regard to the relationship between OCs and cervical dysplasia and carcinoma in situ

- The risk of invasive cervical cancer may be elevated with long duration (>5 years) of OC use

- Present evidence is insufficient to warrant any change in prescribing habits

- Cervical cancer is strongly related to sexually transmitted disease infection, particularly HPV

- Women at risk of STDs should be encouraged to use latex condoms in addition to OCs

- All sexually active women should receive periodic Pap smears

- The frequency of Pap smear screening continues to be debated—ACOG and the American Cancer Society suggest annual screenings

- The US Preventive Services Task Force recommends screening at least once every 3 years; the interval should be determined by the clinician based on the woman's risk factors

---

References

1. Swan SH, Petitti DB. A review of problems of bias and confounding in epidemiologic studies of cervical neoplasia and oral contraceptive use. *Am J Epidemiol* 1982;115:10-18.

2. Slattery ML, Overall JC Jr., Abbott TM, et al. Sexual activity, contraception, genital infections, and cervical cancer: support for a sexually transmitted disease hypothesis. *Am J Epidemiol* 1989;130:248-258.

3. Berget A. Relation of dysplasia and carcinoma of the uterine cervix to age at onset of sexual life and number of coital partners. *Dan Med Bull* 1978;25:172-176.

4. Schiffman MH, Bauer HM, Hoover RN, et al. Epidemiologic evidence showing that human papillomavirus infection causes most cervical intraepithelial neoplasia. *J Natl Cancer Inst* 1993;85:958-964.

5. Kjaer SK, van den Brule AJ, Bock JE, et al. Human papillomavirus—the most significant risk determinant of cervical intraepithelial neoplasia. *Int J Cancer* 1996;65:601-606.

6. Parazzini F, La Vecchia C, Negri E, et al. Reproductive factors and the risk of invasive and intraepithelial cervical neoplasia. *Br J Cancer* 1989;59:805-809.

7. Winkelstein W Jr. Smoking and cervical cancer—current status: a review. *Am J Epidemiol* 1990;131:945-957.

8. Schlesselman JJ. Cancer of the breast and reproductive tract in relation to use of oral contraceptives. *Contraception* 1989;40:1-38.

9. Celentano DD, Klassen AC, Weisman CS, et al. The role of contraceptive use in cervical cancer: the Maryland cervical cancer case-control study. *Am J Epidemiol* 1987;126:592-604.

10. Irwin KL, Rosero-Bixby L, Oberle MW, et al. Oral contraceptives and cervical cancer risk in Costa Rica: detection bias or causal association? *JAMA* 1988; 259:59-64.

11. Beral V, Hannaford P, Kay C. Oral contraceptive use and malignancies of the genital tract. Results from the Royal College of General Practitioners' Oral Contraception Study. *Lancet* 1988;2:1331-1335.

12. Brinton LA, Huggins GR, Lehman HF, et al. Long-term use of oral contraceptives and risk of invasive cervical cancer. *Int J Cancer* 1986:38:339-344.

13. Brinton LA, Reeves WC, Brenes MM, et al. Oral contraceptive use and risk of invasive cervical cancer. *Int J Epidemiol* 1990;19:4-11.

14. WHO Collaborative Study of Neoplasia and Steroid Contraceptives. Invasive cervical cancer and combined oral contraceptives. *BMJ* 1985;290:961-965.

15. WHO Collaborative Study of Neoplasia and Steroid Contraceptives. Invasive squamous-cell cervical carcinoma and combined oral contraceptives: results from a multinational study. *Int J Cancer* 1993;55:228-236.

16. Thomas DB, Ray RM, and The World Health Organization Collaborative Study of Neoplasia and Steroid Contraceptives. Oral contraceptives and invasive adenocarcinomas and adenosquamous carcinomas of the uterine cervix. *Am J Epidemiol* 1996;144:281-189.

17. Zondervan KT, Carpenter LM, Painter R, et al. Oral contraceptives and cervical cancer—further findings from the Oxford Family Planning Association contraceptive study. *Br J Cancer* 1996;73:1291-1297.

18. Ursin G, Pike MC, Preston-Martin S, et al. Sexual, reproductive, and other risk factors for adenocarcinoma of the cervix: results from a population-based case-control study. *Cancer Causes Control* 1996;7:391-401.

2.4: Liver Cancer

The most recent population-based data argue against an association between oral contraceptives and liver cancer. Data indicate no increase in mortality from liver cancer among women in five developed nations. Reassuringly, data from two studies in developing countries, including a large World Health Organization study, also do not support an increased risk of liver cancer with OC use.

Although previous case-control studies have indicated an increased risk of liver cancer with high-dose OC use, more recent epidemiologic data have not confirmed this association. Nine case-control investigations in Western developed nations have found an elevated risk of liver cancer associated with OCs.[1-9] The risks ranged from about two to 20 times the risk for users versus nonusers. Some investigations also have found a higher risk with longer duration of use.[10]

One limitation of all studies of liver cancer among young women, however, is small numbers. Liver cancer among women of reproductive age is rare in developed nations. For example, one case-control study in Catalonia, Spain, reported a borderline statistically significant association between OCs and liver cancer from only six women exposed to OCs and three controls.[6]

Another limitation concerns hepatitis B virus (HBV) infection. Infection with HBV is an important risk factor for primary liver cancer. HBV infection remains endemic in many developing countries, although among developed nations the incidence is low. This risk factor has been overlooked in many studies of the relationship between OCs and liver cancer. Other risk factors for liver cancer include alcohol use, cigarette smoking, and higher parity.

Developing Nations

World Health Organization data from eight developing nations show no increased risk of liver cancer with OC use.[11] WHO researchers found no elevated risk for OC users compared with never users (RR=0.7; 95% CI, 0.4-1.2). In addition, they observed no consistent trend in risk with months of use or time since first or last use.

Developed Countries

If OCs increase the risk of liver cancer, this should be reflected in vital statistics; however, no association is borne out by population mortality data from developed countries. For example, mortality trends from primary liver cancer in England and Wales between 1975 and 1992 indicate that liver cancer mortality has remained constant in women in the age groups that have had major exposure to OCs.[12]

Large cohort studies also do not find an increased risk of liver cancer with OC use. Follow-up data after 20 years from the Oxford Family Planning Association revealed only one death from angiosarcoma—in a woman who did not take OCs.[13] In addition, the Nurses' Health Study reported 10 deaths from liver cancer by 12 years of follow-up. Ever use of OCs was not related to liver cancer mortality (RR=0.4; 95% CI, 0.1-2.4).[14]

Vital statistics from the United States, Sweden, and Japan also cast doubt upon the association between OCs and liver cancer.[15] "Despite several hundred million woman-years of exposure to OCs, women's mortality rates from primary liver cancer have not changed appreciably in the United States. ...despite 3 decades of OC use with prescription sales of up to 70 million cycles per year, women's mortality rates from hepatocellular carcinoma and other primary liver neoplasms have not changed appreciably since hormonal contraception was introduced (Figure 20). In contrast, primary liver cancer mortality rates in men have increased gradually in recent years."[15]

Thus, the population data actually argue *against* an association between OC exposure and liver cancer. According to the researchers, "This analysis of vital statistics from three countries suggests no temporal association between the introduction of OCs and primary liver cancer. The putative increase in risk of two- to 20-fold should have been reflected in vital statistics for this deadly cancer over the past 3 decades."

In addition, new data from the Multicentre International Liver Tumor Study, a large, case-control study conducted in six European nations, found no significant association of OC use with primary liver cancer (OR=0.8; 95% CI, 0.5-1.0).[16] No significant association was found with duration of use or when only hospital or population controls were examined.

Figure 20

Mortality Rates from Primary Liver Cancer According to Gender, United States, 1962-1988, and Annual Sales of Oral Contraceptives, United States, 1964-1988

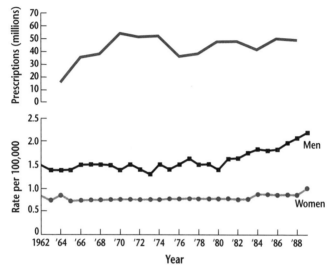

Source: Waetjen LE, Grimes DA. Oral contraceptives and primary liver cancer: temporal trends in three countries. Obstet Gynecol *1996;88:945-949. Reproduced with permission from the American College of Obstetricians and Gynecologists.*

Take Home Messages

- *Liver cancer is rare among reproductive age women in the United States*

- *Vital statistics from developed nations show no increase in liver cancer associated with OC use*

- *Any impact of OCs on liver cancer in US women is negligible*

References

1. Yu MC, Tong MJ, Govindarajan S, et al. Nonviral risk factors for hepatocellular carcinoma in a low-risk population, the non-Asians of Los Angeles County, California. *J Natl Cancer Inst* 1991;83:1820-1826.

2. Henderson BE, Preston-Martin S, Edmondson HA, et al. Hepatocellular carcinoma and oral contraceptives. *Br J Cancer* 1983;48:437-440.

3. Neuberger J, Forman D, Doll R, et al. Oral contraceptives and hepatocellular carcinoma. *BMJ* (Clin Res Ed) 1986;292:1355-1357.

4. Forman D, Vincent TJ, Doll R. Cancer of the liver and the use of oral contraceptives. *BMJ* (Clin Res Ed) 1986;292:1357-1361.

5. La Vecchia C, Negri E, Parazzini F. Oral contraceptives and primary liver cancer. *Br J Cancer* 1989;59:460-461.

6. Vall-Mayans MV, Calvet X, Bruix J, et al. Risk factors for hepatocellular carcinoma in Catalonia, Spain. *Int J Cancer* 1990;46:378-381.

7. Palmer JR, Rosenberg L, Kaufman DW, et al. Oral contraceptive use and liver cancer. *Am J Epidemiol* 1989;130:878-882.

8. Hsing AW, Hoover RN, McLaughlin JK, et al. Oral contraceptives and primary liver cancer among young women. *Cancer Causes Control* 1992;3:43-48.

9. Tavani A, Negri E, Parazzini F, et al. Female hormone utilisation and risk of hepatocellular carcinoma. *Br J Cancer* 1993;67:635-637.

10. Prentice RL. Epidemiologic data on exogenous hormones and hepatocellular carcinoma and selected other cancers. *Prev Med* 1991;20:38-46.

11. WHO Collaborative Study of Neoplasia and Steroid Contraceptives. Combined oral contraceptives and liver cancer. *Int J Cancer* 1989;43:254-259.

12. Mant JWF, Vessey MP. Trends in mortality from primary liver cancer in England and Wales 1975-92: influence of oral contraceptives. *Br J Cancer* 1995;72:800-803.

13. Vessey MP, Villard-Mackintosh L, McPherson K, et al. Mortality among oral contraceptive users: 20 year follow-up of women in a cohort study. *BMJ* 1989;299:1487-1491.

14. Colditz GA. Oral contraceptive use and mortality during 12 years of follow-up: the Nurses' Health Study. *Ann Intern Med* 1994;120:821-826.

15. Waetjen LE, Grimes DA. Oral contraceptives and primary liver cancer: temporal trends in three countries. *Obstet Gynecol* 1996;88:945-949.

16. The Collaborative MILTS Project Team. Oral contraceptives and liver cancer. *Contraception* 1997;56:275-284.

2.5: Benign Gallbladder Disease

Studies conducted in the 1970s suggested that high-dose combination oral contraceptive use was associated with an increased risk of gallbladder disease.[1,2] A meta-analysis of studies published through 1990, however, found only nine that had rigorous methods. The investigators pooled the results of these nine and found a slightly elevated risk with current OC use; however, the latest data from two large cohort studies, the Royal College of General Practitioners' (RCGP) Oral Contraception Study and the Oxford Family Planning Association (FPA) Study, indicate the risk estimate has decreased with subsequent analyses and use of low-dose OCs. In fact, the Oxford FPA's latest findings suggest no increased risk of gallbladder disease with low-dose OC use.

How oral contraceptives might influence gallbladder disease is unclear. Researchers have hypothesized that exogenous steroids may increase biliary cholesterol saturation and/or decrease gallbladder motility. These may, in turn, increase formation of gallstones or cause gallbladder inflammation. Early studies suggested an association between OCs and both these conditions.

Product Labeling vs Current Data

Oral contraceptive product labeling remains outdated. The product literature states, "Studies report an increased risk of surgically confirmed gallbladder disease in users of oral contraceptives and estrogens." However, the FDA-approved package labeling cites three references, all of which refer to data prior to 1975. In addition, two of the references have risks whose 95% confidence limits include 1.0, which means they did not reach statistical significance.

New analyses suggest either no increased risk of gallbladder disease or, at most, a small, transitory increased risk with current use.[3,4] The small risk could be due to bias or chance, however. A causal relationship is clinically improbable because gallstones take many years to develop. Pooled data suggest that OC use may enhance the development of symptoms from existing gallstones.

A meta-analysis of epidemiologic studies of gallbladder disease (excluding gallbladder cancer) and OC use found nine with rigorous methods.[5] These nine had similar findings of about a 30% to 40% increased risk of gallbladder disease with OC use; however, none of the findings were statistically significant. On the other hand, the overall odds ratio of 1.4 (95% CI, 1.2-1.6) reached statistical significance. The meta-analysis also found evidence to suggest a dose-effect relationship with lower-dose preparations having less of an effect.

Data from the two large United Kingdom cohort studies have shown progressively lower risk estimates with subsequent follow-up. The results from RCGP in 1994 yielded a nonsignificant relative risk of gallbladder disease for users of OCs compared to never users of 1.2 (95% CI, 1.0-1.3)[3]; risks were 1.3 (95% CI, 1.0-1.8) in 1974 and 1.1 (95% CI, 1.0-1.3) in 1982. On the other hand, RCGP data indicate that cigarette smoking and parity increase the risk of gallbladder disease.

The Oxford FPA shows a similar trend of lower risk estimates with longer follow-up (Figure 21).[4] In 1994, the researchers reported no significant increased risk of gallbladder disease with OC use compared to never use (RR=1.1; 95% CI, 0.9-1.3). The analysis included 482 women with benign gallbladder disease, which was surgically confirmed in 407 women.

Figure 21

Risk of Gallbladder Disease with Oral Contraceptive Use, Oxford Family Planning Association Study— 1976, 1982, and 1994

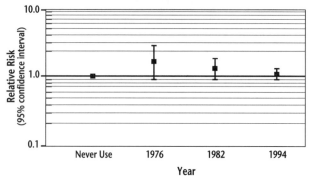

Source: Adapted from references 2, 4, and 6.

In addition, no relationship was found between duration of use and risk. After 97 months or more of use compared to never use, women's relative risk of developing benign gallbladder disease was 1.1 (95% CI, 0.8-1.5). The researchers also looked at the possible interaction between gallbladder disease, OC use, and body mass index or age. They again found no indication of any increased risk of disease with OC use and either of these factors. On the other hand, the Oxford FPA found significantly elevated risks of gall-bladder disease with parity, cigarette smoking, and Quetelets Index (a measure of body mass) similar to previously reported findings.[6]

Take Home Messages

■ *Recent data suggest no increased risk of benign gallbladder disease with low-dose OC use*

■ *Long-term OC use does not appear to confer any added risk*

References

1. Royal College of General Practitioners. *Oral Contraceptives and Health.* London: Pitman Medical; 1974:57-59.

2. Vessey M, Doll R, Peto R, et al. A long-term follow-up study of women using different methods of contraception—an interim report. *J Biosoc Sci* 1976;8: 373-427.

3. Murray FE, Logan RFA, Hannaford PC, et al. Cigarette smoking and parity as risk factors for the development of symptomatic gallbladder disease in women: results of the Royal College of General Practitioners' oral contraception study. *Gut* 1994;35:107-111.

4. Vessey M, Painter R. Oral contraceptive use and benign gallbladder disease; revisited. *Contraception* 1994;50:167-173.

5. Thijs C, Knipschild P. Oral contraceptives and the risk of gallbladder disease: a meta-analysis. *Am J Public Health* 1993;83:1113-1120.

6. Layde PM, Vessey MP, Yeates D. Risk factors for gall-bladder disease: a cohort study of young women attending family planning clinics. *J Epidemiol Community Health* 1982;36:274-278.

2.6: Sickle Cell Disease

Women with sickle cell disease and their fetuses are at high risk of complications. Therefore, highly effective contraception is desirable, and the benefits of oral contraceptives generally outweigh the risks.

Sickle cell hemoglobinopathies are caused by a genetic mutation that causes a deformity in the hemoglobin of red blood cells. The recessive autosomal gene is common in indigenous populations in areas where malaria is endemic. The presence of sickle cell trait (heterozygous [HbAS]) makes the carrier more resistant to malaria, an advantage in equatorial Africa and other areas where malaria is widespread. Those who inherit the trait from both parents (homozygous [HbSS]) have sickle cell anemia, a serious condition characterized by painful clustering of abnormal red blood cells.

In persons with sickle cell disease, abnormal hemoglobin precipitates and becomes rigid when subjected to oxygen deprivation. The erythrocyte membranes are rendered fragile and deform into a sickle shape. Although one early hypothesis suggested that the thrombotic episodes in patients with sickle cell anemia were due to hormonal influences, this has never been proven.

The etiology differs between thrombotic episodes in women with sickle cell disease and those using OCs.[1,2] For women with sickle cell anemia, hypoxia precipitates the sickling phenomenon, which results in clustering of abnormally shaped red blood cells and occlusion of blood vessels.[2,3] No known mechanism explains how OCs could cause hypoxia and exacerbate sickling crises.

Sickling crises can be precipitated by infection, pregnancy, and other factors, such as emotional stress, alcohol, and menstrual periods, but the latter mechanisms are not well understood. Whether OCs may foster sickling remains a theoretical, but unproven, concern. The theoretical concern is based on the belief that an additive risk could ensue when two clotting processes (erythrocyte clustering in sicklers and clotting changes induced by OCs) coincide. Whether any alterations in clotting parameters caused by OCs work synergistically with sickle cell clustering is unknown. In fact, modern, low-dose OC preparations have minimal demonstrable impact on clotting factors.

The evidence concerning adverse effects is too weak and the risks of pregnancy too high to deny OCs to women with sickle cell disease.[1,2,4-6] Pregnancy carries increased risks of complications for women and is associated with spontaneous abortion, intrauterine growth restriction, and higher neonatal mortality.[3]

OC Users with Sickle Cell Disease

Data are limited concerning the use of OCs in women with sickle cell anemia. No prospective cohort or case-control investigations have examined the suggested association between OCs and thrombotic phenomena in women with sickle cell hemoglobinopathies. Small observational studies found no evidence that women with sickle cell disease face higher risks because of OC use.[7-9] Additional studies among black women offer little support for a synergistic effect of OCs on sickle cell disease.[10,11] A recent, small observational study (n=30) found no difference in red blood cell deformability (as measured by clogging rate and red cell transit time) among women using combination OCs, progestin-only OCs, and nonhormonal methods.[12]

The World Health Organization gives sickle cell disease a "2" rating, which means that, in general, the benefits from the use of oral contraceptives generally outweigh the risks for women with the disease.[5] Sickle cell trait presents no contraindication to OC use. Members of an international workshop came to similar conclusions.[6]

 Injectable contraception remains the first choice for women with sickle cell disease because it reduces the frequency of sickling crises[13]; however, women who cannot or do not wish to use depot medroxyprogesterone acetate (DMPA) or other methods of birth control should not be prohibited from using OCs.

Take Home Messages

- The benefits of OC use generally outweigh the risks for women with sickle cell disease

- Available data from small observational studies of women with sickle cell disease using OCs indicate no increased risk of sickling crises or thromboembolic events

- DMPA may be the method of choice because it reduces sickling crises

---

References

1. Goldzieher JW, Zamah NM. Oral contraceptive side effects: where's the beef? *Contraception* 1995;52:327-335.

2. Freie HMP. Sickle cell diseases and hormonal contraception. *Acta Obstet Gynecol Scand* 1983;62:211-217.

3. Charache S, Niebyl JR. Pregnancy in sickle cell disease. *Clin Haematol* 1985; 14:729-746.

4. Vichinsky E, McDonald C. Letter to the editor. *J Adolesc Health Care* 1988; 9:87.

5. Family and Reproductive Health Programme. *Improving Access to Quality Care in Family Planning. Medical Eligibility Criteria for Contraceptive Use.* Geneva: World Health Organization; 1996:1-30.

6. Hannaford PC, Webb AMC. Evidence-guided prescribing of combined oral contraceptives: consensus statement. *Contraception* 1996;54:125-129.

7. Lutcher CL. Blood coagulation studies and the effect of oral contraceptives in patients with sickle cell anemia. *Clin Res* 1976;24:47A. Abstract.

8. Lutcher CL, Harris P, Henderson PA, et al. A lack of morbidity from oral contraception in women with sickle cell anemia. *Clin Res* 1981;29:863A. Abstract.

9. Lutcher CL, Milner PF. Contraceptive-induced vascular occlusive events in sickle cell disorders—fact or fiction? *Clin Res* 1986;34:217A. Abstract.

10. Herson J, Sharma S, Crocker CL, et al. Physical complaints of patients with sickle cell trait. *J Reprod Med* 1975;14:129-132.

11. Blumstein BA, Douglas MB, Hall WD. Blood pressure changes and oral contraceptive use: a study of 2676 black women in the southeastern United States. *Am J Epidemiol* 1980;112:529-532.

12. Yoong WC, Tuck SM, Yardumian A. Red cell deformability in oral contraceptive pill users with sickle cell anaemia. *Br J Haematol* 1999;104:868-870.

13. De Ceulaer K, Gruber C, Hayes R, et al. Medroxyprogesterone acetate and homozygous sickle cell disease. *Lancet* 1982;ii:229-231.

2.7: Epilepsy

Oral contraceptives may be used for contraception in women with epilepsy. The condition is not a concern; however, certain anticonvulsants (phenytoin, phenobarbital, carbamazepine, primidone, and ethosuximide) induce hepatic enzymes, enhance the metabolism of sex hormones, and can reduce OC efficacy.[1-4] WHO notes that drug interactions may result in a higher-risk pregnancy (due to the teratogenic effects of anticonvulsants) and suggests long-term users of these anticonvulsants may wish to use another highly effective method of birth control.[5]

OCs generally do not exacerbate seizures in women with epilepsy.[1,4] Pharmacokinetic data and case reports (52 by 1983), however, have linked the use of certain antiepileptic agents with decreased sex steroid metabolism and reports of unintended pregnancy.[1,2,4,6] The induction of hepatic enzymes may affect the metabolism of both estrogen and progestin, although the degree of increased metabolism is highly variable.

Based on these data, clinicians traditionally have been advised to consider using a high-dose estrogen OC for women with epilepsy taking these anticonvulsants. Importantly, however, because the estrogen and progestin work synergistically to provide the contraceptive effect, progestin pharmacokinetics also play a role in maintaining contraceptive protection. Some data indicate, for example, that the contraceptive efficacy of levonorgestrel can be hampered by anticonvulsants in women using contraceptive implants.[7,8]

Because both sex hormones may be affected, clinicians may wish to choose a high-dose estrogen OC. In addition, progestin pharmacokinetics suggest using an OC containing a progestin with minimal first-pass metabolism to ensure maximum bioavailability and contraceptive effect.

On the other hand, epileptic women now have more anticonvulsant options, which make using OCs more effective. For example, sodium valproate and newer antiepileptics, such as gabapentin, lamotrigine, and felbamate, do not induce hepatic enzymes. Women using these drugs can safely use low-dose OCs.

A small study found that injectable medroxyprogesterone acetate reduced seizures.[9] For this reason, DMPA is an appealing contraceptive method for this population.[1,4]

Take Home Messages

- *Epileptic women choosing to use combination OCs may need a higher-dose OC if they use medications that induce hepatic enzymes*

- *Pharmacokinetic data suggest using an OC containing a progestin with minimal first-pass metabolism in order to achieve the greatest bioavailability and maintain adequate contraceptive protection*

- *The exact dosage is impossible to predict, due to individual variations in metabolism*

- *DMPA can reduce seizure frequency, making it an appealing contraceptive choice for this population*

References

1. Mattson RH, Cramer JA, Darney PD, et al. Use of oral contraceptives by women with epilepsy. *JAMA* 1986;256:238-240.

2. Back DJ, Orme MLE. Pharmacokinetic drug interactions with oral contraceptives. *Clin Pharmacokinet* 1990;18:472-484.

3. Goldzieher JW. *Hormonal Contraception: Pills, Injections & Implants.* 4th ed. Ontario: EMIS-CANADA; 1994:52-57.

4. Mattson RH, Rebar RW. Contraceptive methods for women with neurologic disorders. *Am J Obstet Gynecol* 1993;168:2027-2032.

5. Family and Reproductive Health Programme. *Improving Access to Quality Care in Family Planning. Medical Eligibility Criteria for Contraceptive Use.* Geneva: World Health Organization; 1996:1-30.

6. Sonnen AE. Sodium valproate and the contraceptive pill. *Br J Clin Pract Symp* 1983;27(suppl):31-36.

7. Odlind V, Olsson SE. Enhanced metabolism of levonorgestrel during phenytoin treatment in a woman with Norplant implants. *Contraception* 1986;33:257-261.

8. Haukkamaa M. Contraception by NORPLANT® capsules is not reliable in epileptic patients on anticonvulsant treatment. *Contraception* 1986;33:559-565.

9. Mattson RH, Cramer JA, Caldwell BV, et al. Treatment of seizures with medroxyprogesterone acetate: preliminary report. *Neurology* 1984;34:1255-1258.

2.8: Liver Disease

How the small quantities of sex steroids in oral contraceptives may affect a diseased liver is unknown. However, because contraceptive steroids are metabolized by the liver, active liver disease is generally considered a contraindication to the use of oral contraceptives.[1,2]

WHO notes that combination OCs may adversely affect women whose liver function is already compromised.[3] Active viral hepatitis and severe cirrhosis (decompensated) generally preclude the use of OCs, although one study of six women with chronic inflammatory hepatitis found significantly improved liver enzymes during treatment with 20 µg ethinyl estradiol.[4]

In a woman with mild liver dysfunction, the benefits of OCs may outweigh the risks. A history of jaundice of pregnancy suggests caution; however, an assessment of the risks and benefits is warranted, as pregnancy carries a much greater risk of high estrogen exposure.[2] Therapeutic use of OCs may be considered for women with transient liver dysfunction (eg, suppression of menses in women receiving chemotherapy). Asymptomatic hepatitis carriers may use oral contraceptives.

Take Home Messages

- *Women with active liver disease generally should avoid combination OCs for contraception*
- *Asymptomatic hepatitis carriers may use OCs*
- *Clinicians should weigh the potential benefits vs risks in women with mild liver impairment*
- *Liver tumors, extremely rare among women of reproductive age, preclude the use of OCs*

References

1. Orme ML, Back DJ, Breckenridge AM. Clinical pharmacokinetics of oral contraceptive steroids. *Clin Pharmacokin* 1983;8:95-136.

2. Goldzieher JW. *Hormonal Contraception: Pills, Injections & Implants.* 4th ed. Ontario: EMIS-CANADA; 1998:216-223.

3. Family and Reproductive Health Programme. *Improving Access to Quality Care in Family Planning. Medical Eligibility Criteria for Contraceptive Use.* Geneva: World Health Organization; 1996:1-30.

4. Guattery JM, Faloon WW, Biery DL. Effect of ethinyl estradiol on chronic active hepatitis. *Ann Intern Med* 1997;126:88. Letter.

2.9: Headache/Migraine

The World Health Organization's revised medical eligibility criteria suggest that headaches have been used too frequently to deny women oral contraceptives. WHO recommends that women with serious migraine that includes focal neurological symptoms be cautioned against using OCs.[1] In general, the benefits of OC use outweigh the risks for women who have common migraine (no aura). Clinicians need to take the presence of other stroke risk factors into consideration, however, and monitor women for changes in the frequency or severity of headaches.

The origin of the concern regarding OCs and headaches dates back to early studies of the pill. Because stroke may be preceded by headache, clinicians questioned whether prescribing OCs for women with headaches could precipitate a stroke. Importantly, screening for such risk factors as smoking and hypertension, as well as using low-dose pills, has greatly reduced the risk of vascular complications in OC users.[2-4] The latest evidence suggests that healthy, nonsmoking women of reproductive age using low-dose OCs (≤35 μg estrogen) have no significantly increased risk of stroke.[5-7]

At the initial visit, clinicians should try to determine which type(s) of headache the patient has experienced in the past, and the frequency and severity of the problem. Certain symptoms are indicative of a particular headache, although patients may experience more than one type of headache (Table 16). Patients may not be clear about the type of headache they have. The word *migraine* is often used by patients simply to describe a bad headache, which can create confusion. A thorough headache history and family history should be taken to help with the differential diagnosis.

Reassure women that headaches are reported by only a small percentage of women using OCs, and that many users report improvement in headaches. For example, one randomized, triple-blind investigation of 124 women using a low-dose OC found that after 1 month of use, 48% of women reported no change in nonmigrainous headaches, 48% reported fewer headaches, and only 4% reported an increase in headaches.[8] Reassurance is important, as worsening headaches can lead to quitting OCs in teens, whatever the cause.[9]

Table 16

Symptoms of Tension Headache

- Occur sporadically
- Steady, dull ache
- Relief with aspirin or acetaminophen
- Often associated with stress, anxiety, fatigue, or anger
- Tense shoulder/neck muscles

Symptoms of Migraine without Aura (Common Migraine)

- Throbbing or pulsating unilateral pain
- Sensitivity to light or sound
- Not easily relieved by aspirin or acetaminophen
- Nausea/vomiting/anorexia
- May be triggered by food, alcohol
- May be related to onset of menses
- Often a family history of migraine headache

Symptoms of Migraine with Aura (Classic Migraine)

(Same symptoms as common migraine, plus additional neurologic disturbances)

- Visual aura that may include jagged or wavy lines, dots or flashing lights, or tunnel vision
- May have neurological symptoms during, but not after, headache

Symptoms Suggesting Intracranial Pathology

- Neurological symptoms during and after headache
- "Worst headache of my life"
- Increased blood pressure
- Loss of consciousness
- Headache wakes patient from sleep

Types of Headaches

Several types of headaches are common: tension headaches, migraine without aura (common migraine), and migraine with aura (classic migraine). Less common are cluster headaches, post-traumatic headaches, headaches associated with vascular disorders (such as stroke, hematoma, and hypertension), and headaches arising from intracranial pathology.[10] Making the distinction among migraine with aura, migraine without aura, and tension headache is important because each type of headache suggests different contraceptive management.

Tension Headache

The most common type of headache is muscle contraction or tension headache. Tension headache may be associated with depression, anxiety, emotional upset, or stress and is characterized by bilateral pain and a tight, band-like sensation. Often, the neck and shoulder muscles are tight and painful. Patients usually describe the pain as a dull, steady ache. Importantly, no neurological deficits occur and the pain may be alleviated by aspirin, acetaminophen, nonsteroidal anti-inflammatories, or muscle relaxants. Tension headache presents no contraindication to OC use.

Migraine Headache

Migraine headaches are typically recurrent episodes of throbbing or pulsating pain, usually accompanied by nausea, vomiting, or anorexia. Frequently, the patient reports a family history of migraine; the majority of sufferers are women by an approximate 2:1 ratio.[11]

The etiology of migraine is not fully understood. Many patients report that fatigue, bright light, missing meals, certain foods or beverages (aged cheese or alcohol, for example), and changes in the weather can trigger migraine episodes. A hormonal mechanism may be involved; many women report that migraine episodes are linked to their menstrual cycle.[12] *Menstrual migraine* describes a migraine that occurs prior to or during menstruation, but not at other times. Falling levels of female sex hormones may trigger a migraine with onset of menses or during the hormone-free interval of OCs (estrogen-withdrawal migraine).

Little evidence exists to support a relationship between OCs and an increased risk or exacerbation of migraine.[13] A Hungarian study of women with menstrual migraine headaches found that some headaches worsened, but many improved or stopped altogether.[14] (For further discussion of using OCs to treat menstrual migraine, see the section on treatment of medical disorders.)

Migraine without Aura

Migraine without aura is seen more frequently in the general population than classic migraine. Migraine without aura is not accompanied by focal neurological symptoms.

Migraine with Aura

Migraine with aura is characterized by unilateral, throbbing pain accompanied by prodromal symptoms that occur just prior to or during the attack, usually developing over 5 to 20 minutes and lasting less than 60 minutes.[10-12] Focal neurological deficits, such as visual disturbances, are present. These include depressed or absent areas within the visual field, flashing lights or spots, or zigzag lines. Unilateral weakness or numbness, dizziness, and sensitivity to light or sound can also occur. Importantly, however, the neurological symptoms resolve when the headache subsides.

Migraine, OCs, and Risk of Stroke

Studies of stroke have identified migraine, particularly migraine with aura, as an independent risk factor for stroke among reproductive age women.[15-22] Migraine can be considered both a direct cause and a remote risk factor.[11] The International Headache Society terms an attack of migraine complicated by stroke as *migrainous infarction.*[10]

New data from the World Health Organization indicate a link between migraine and ischemic stroke, but not hemorrhagic stroke.[17] The WHO study found a significant increased risk of ischemic stroke among women who experienced migraine with aura (OR=3.8; 95% CI, 1.3-11.5). In addition, the WHO investigation found an increased, but nonsignificant, risk of stroke in women reporting migraine without aura (OR=3.0; 95% CI, 0.7-14.0). Substantially elevated odds ratios occurred when women with migraine also had high blood pressure or smoked cigarettes. A family history of migraine was associated with a five times greater risk of ischemic stroke (OR=5.0; 95% CI, 2.0-12.3). The WHO study estimated that 20% to 40% of strokes in migrainous women developed directly out of a migraine attack.

WHO also evaluated the relationship among migraine, use of OCs, and stroke.[17] Among women reporting migraine but not using OCs, the odds ratio for ischemic stroke was 2.3 (95% CI, 0.7-7.5). Among women reporting migraine using low-dose OCs, the odds ratio of ischemic stroke was higher, 6.6 (95% CI, 0.8-54.8), but did not reach statistical significance. By contrast, migrainous women who also smoked cigarettes had a significant risk of ischemic stroke (OR=7.4; 95% CI, 2.1-25.5). In addition, a family history of migraine had a strong effect on the likelihood of ischemic stroke. Women with a family history of migraine were 17 times more likely to experience ischemic stroke compared to women with no family history of migraine (OR=17.3; 95% CI, 4.4-67.2).

Data on how OC use affects migraines suggested little impact on frequency or severity. For example, 82% and 88% of women experiencing either ischemic or hemorrhagic stroke, respectively, reported no change in the frequency of headache after beginning OC use. In addition, 84% of women with ischemic and 92% of women with hemorrhagic stroke reported that OC use had no effect on the type of migraine they experienced. In other words, OCs were not likely to change migraine without aura into migraine with aura.

Because the WHO investigation found a threefold, but non-significant, risk of ischemic stroke among women reporting migraine without aura, debate has ensued concerning OC clinical practice guidelines.[23-27] In general, the benefits of OCs for women who experience migraine without aura outweigh the risks. The UK Family Planning Association revised its recommendations for clinical practice with regard to the use of OCs in women with migraine.[23] Their guidelines state that the advantages of combination OCs generally outweigh the risks as long as a woman has no additional risk factors for stroke (WHO Category 2). The UK guidelines, however, suggest a WHO Category 3 (risks generally outweigh the benefits) for women who experience migraine without aura if they have one additional risk factor for stroke. These risk factors include age 35 years or older, diabetes mellitus, hyperlipidemia, hypertension, obesity (body mass index >30), family history of arterial disease ≤45 years, and smoking cigarettes. The UK Family Planning Association suggests a WHO Category 4 (should not use) in women who experience migraine without aura if more than one additional risk factor for stroke is present. The agency also suggests that the lowest estrogen dose OC be used for women who experience migraine.

Evaluation of Headaches in OC Users

A worsening of headaches, either in severity or frequency, or the new onset of headaches requires an evaluation (including blood pressure measurement). Headaches that are severe, persistent, or of sudden onset, or abnormal neurological signs that persist after a headache has resolved should be evaluated. These types of headaches may warrant discontinuing OCs, at least temporarily, until the situation is resolved or an alternative diagnosis is made (Table 17). If OCs are discontinued, practitioners should counsel patients about alternative methods of contraception. Progestin-only OCs can be safely used by women with migraine.

Table 17

Headaches Requiring Further Evaluation

- Previously existing migraines that suddenly worsen or change
- Headaches of unusual severity and sudden onset
- Headaches followed by persistent abnormal neurological findings
- Headaches that are much worse when recumbent or with coughing, sneezing, coitus, or Valsalva's maneuver
- Headache that wakes a patient from sleep
- Headaches that begin at an older age without a previous history or positive family history

Source: Adapted from Digre K, 1987, et al (see reference 12).

Take Home Messages

Tension headache

- *Women with tension headache may use OCs*

Migraine without aura

- *The benefits of combination OC use generally outweigh the risks; clinicians may wish to use the lowest-dose estrogen OC*
- *Monitor frequency and severity of headaches during use of OCs*

Continued on next page

> ## *Take Home Messages* (continued)
>
> ■ *Further evaluate and stop OCs if migraine changes to include neurological symptoms, especially double vision or loss of vision*
>
> ■ *Consider prior frequency of headache and presence of other stroke risk factors, such as age, cigarette smoking, and hypertension, when counseling patient about options*
>
> ### Migraine with aura
>
> ■ *Women who experience migraine with focal neurological symptoms should avoid use of OCs, but the risk-to-benefit ratio must be weighed in cases where a high-risk pregnancy could result*
>
> ■ *Progestin-only OCs can be safely used by women with migraine*

References

1. Family and Reproductive Health Programme. *Improving Access to Quality Care in Family Planning. Medical Eligibility Criteria for Contraceptive Use.* Geneva: World Health Organization; 1996:1-30.

2. Croft P, Hannaford PC. Risk factors for acute myocardial infarction in women: evidence from the Royal College of General Practitioners' oral contraception study. *BMJ* 1989;298:165-168.

3. Stampfer MJ, Willett WC, Colditz GA, et al. Past use of oral contraceptives and cardiovascular disease: a meta-analysis in the context of the Nurses' Health Study. *Am J Obstet Gynecol* 1990;163:285-291.

4. Porter JB, Hunter JR, Jick H, et al. Oral contraceptives and nonfatal vascular disease. *Obstet Gynecol* 1985;66:1-4.

5. Petitti DB, Sidney S, Bernstein A, et al. Stroke in users of low-dose oral contraceptives. *N Engl J Med* 1996;335:8-15.

6. WHO Collaborative Study of Cardiovascular Disease and Steroid Hormone Contraception. Ischaemic stroke and combined oral contraceptives: results of an international, multicentre, case-control study. *Lancet* 1996;348:498-505.

7. WHO Collaborative Study of Cardiovascular Disease and Steroid Hormone Contraception. Haemorrhagic stroke, overall stroke risk, and combined oral contraceptives: results of an international, multicentre, case-control study. *Lancet* 1996;348:505-510.

8. Villegas-Salas E, Ponce de Leon R, Juarez-Perez MA, et al. Effect of vitamin B_6 on the side effects of a low-dose combined oral contraceptive. *Contraception* 1997;55:245-248.

9. Emans SJ, Grace E, Woods ER, et al. Adolescents' compliance with the use of oral contraceptives. *JAMA* 1987;257:3377-3381.

10. International Headache Society. Classification and diagnostic criteria for headache disorders, cranial neuralgias and facial pain. *Cephalalgia* 1988;8 (suppl 7):1-96.

11. Tietjen GE. The relationship of migraine and stroke. *Neuroepidemiology* 2000;19:13-19.

12. Digre K, Damasio H. Menstrual migraine: differential diagnosis, evaluation and treatment. *Clin Obstet Gynecol* 1987;30:417-430.

13. Benson MD, Rebar RW. Relationship of migraine headache and stroke to oral contraceptive use. *J Reprod Med* 1986;31:1082-1088.

14. Karsay K. The relationship between vascular headaches and low-dose oral contraceptives. *Therapia Hungarica* 1990;38:181-185.

15. Collaborative Group for the Study of Stroke in Young Women. Oral contraceptives and stroke in young women: associated risk factors. *JAMA* 1975;75:718-722.

16. Lidegaard O. Oral contraceptives, pregnancy and the risk of cerebral thromboembolism: the influence of diabetes, hypertension, migraine and previous thrombotic disease. *Br J Obstet Gynaecol* 1995;102:153-159.

17. Chang CL, Donaghy M, Poulter N, et al. Migraine and stroke in young women: case-control study. *BMJ* 1999;318:13-18.

18. Merikangas KR, Fenton BT, Cheng SH, et al. Association between migraine and stroke in a large-scale epidemiological study of the United States. *Arch Neurol* 1997;54:362-368.

19. Schwartz SM, Petitti DB, Siscovick DS, et al. Stroke and use of low-dose oral contraceptives in young women. A pooled analysis of two US studies. *Stroke* 1998;29:2277-2284.

20. Tzourio C, Tehindrazanarivelo A, Iglésias S, et al. Case-control study of migraine and risk of ischaemic stroke in young women. *BMJ* 1995;310:830-833.

21. Marini C, Carolei A, Roberts RS, et al. Focal cerebral ischaemia in young adults; a collaborative case-control study. *Neuroepidemiology* 1993;12:70-71.

22. Carolei A, Marini C, De Matteis G. History of migraine and risk of cerebral ischaemia in young adults. *Lancet* 1996;347:1503-1506.

23. MacGregor EA, Guillebaud J, and the Clinical and Scientific Committee of the Faculty of Family Planning and Reproductive Health Care and the Family Planning Association. Recommendations for clinical practice. Combined oral contraceptives, migraine and ischaemic stroke. *Br J Fam Plann* 1998;24:55-60.

24. Becker WJ. Use of oral contraceptives in patients with migraine. *Neurology* 1999;53(suppl 1):S19-S25.

25. MacGregor EA, Guillebaud J. Authors' results suggest that all types of migraine are contraindications to oral contraceptives. *BMJ* 1999;318:1485. Letter.

26. Olesen J. Prospective study is needed to determine what clinical practice in migraine should be. *BMJ* 1999;318:1485. Letter.

27. Donaghy M, Poulter NR, Chang CL. Authors' reply. *BMJ* 1999;318:1485. Letter.

2.10: Drug Interactions

The possible interaction of oral contraceptives with other drugs has been the subject of numerous case reports since the early 1970s. Some interactions are well documented and therapeutically relevant; many remain unproven or are the subject of continuing controversy.

Reports of drug interactions with OCs fall into two general categories: the efficacy of oral contraceptive steroids may be affected by concomitant administration of other drugs and oral contraceptives may interfere with the metabolism of other agents. Interference from OCs can either increase or decrease the effectiveness of other drugs. Likewise, OC efficacy may either be impaired or enhanced by concurrent drug therapy; impairment may result in breakthrough bleeding (and, occasionally, pregnancy), while enhancement of oral contraceptive efficacy may increase side effects.

Strong evidence suggests griseofulvin, rifampin, and anticonvulsants that induce hepatic enzymes decrease OC effectiveness. Tables 18 through 20 list interactions between OCs and other drugs, the nature of the interaction, and the strength of the evidence.[1-17]

Anticonvulsants

The enzyme-inducing nature of a number of anticonvulsant drugs may increase the metabolism of OC steroids, resulting in insufficient levels of estrogen or progestin to prevent ovulation. The most commonly implicated anticonvulsant agents are phenobarbital and phenytoin, although carbamazepine, primidone, and ethosuximide have also been suspected of interfering with OC efficacy.[1-3] (For further discussion, see the section on epilepsy.)

Antibiotics

An unproven, but widely accepted, drug interaction involves the effect of antibiotics on OC efficacy. Despite a number of case reports implicating penicillins, tetracyclines, and other antibiotics in causing OC failure, no firm pharmacokinetic evidence links antibiotic administration with altered steroid blood concentrations.[2]

Antibiotics have been postulated to interfere with OC efficacy by altering enterohepatic recirculation. Enterohepatic recirculation occurs when, following conjugation of contraceptive steroids in the liver and upper small intestine, conjugates pass through the bile into the colon. Bacterial enzymes in the colon then deconjugate the agents, which are then reabsorbed, presumably causing an increase in circulating ethinyl estradiol. Data from animal studies indicate that antibiotics can interrupt this process by killing the bacteria responsible for deconjugation in the colon, resulting in decreased hormone levels and reduced contraceptive efficacy.[2,4] Several studies involving human subjects, however, have failed to support such an interaction.

Studies of penicillins have found no association between their use and a decrease in OC efficacy.[6-11] Additionally, two studies have shown no important interactions between oral contraceptives and tetracycline or doxycycline.[12,13]

Furthermore, data suggest no interference from use of fluoro-quinolone antibiotics. A randomized, double-blind, placebo-controlled crossover trial of 24 women treated with ciprofloxacin and a 30 μg EE OC containing desogestrel found no pharmacokinetic interaction between the two drugs. Blood levels of estrogen and progestin indicated no or very little ovarian activity and no ovulation.[15] A similar randomized trial also found no evidence of ovulation during 7-day treatment with ofloxacin among 20 women using a 30 μg EE OC containing levonorgestrel.[16] A small trial of temafloxacin given during day 1 through day 7 of the cycle also found no indication of ovulation.[17]

Some researchers have recommended that patients taking antibiotics use an additional contraceptive method, such as a condom. Instructions concerning how long to use added protection varies.[5] The added precaution of condoms is probably unnecessary for efficacy, but remains important for women at risk of STDs.

Some have suggested that patients on long-term antibiotic therapy, such as oral antibiotics for the treatment of acne, be monitored for breakthrough bleeding, and pill dose be increased or a condom used if spotting occurs.[3] On the other hand, one might expect OC efficacy to stabilize over the course of long-term therapy as bacteria responsible for steroid deconjugation develop a resistance to the antibiotic. Thus, a gradual rise in contraceptive efficacy could follow the postulated initial drop in such patients. Given the huge number of subjects that would be needed for clinical trials addressing these issues, it is unlikely that a definitive answer will emerge.

The antituberculosis drug rifampin, also used for meningitis prophylaxis, decreases OC efficacy. During the early and mid-1970s, numerous pill failures were reported among tuberculosis patients.[2,4] Rifampin has potent enzyme-inducing properties and causes a reduction in both progestin and estrogen levels.[2]

The antifungal drug griseofulvin has been associated with breakthrough bleeding and a small number of pregnancies among OC users.[2,14] Although the drug is known to modify hepatic enzyme activity in mice, evidence of a major enzyme-inducing effect in humans is lacking.[2] Patients using both drugs may require a higher-dose OC to maintain optimum contraceptive efficacy.[3]

Benzodiazepines

Although documentation is not extensive, OC use may affect the activity of some benzodiazepine tranquilizers—either increasing or decreasing their efficacy.

Other Medications

Some evidence indicates that OCs may reduce or potentiate the efficacy of certain analgesics, anti-inflammatories (corticosteroids), bronchodilators, and antihypertensives. No data indicate any interaction between selective serotonin reuptake inhibitors and OCs.

Table 18

Drugs That May Enhance Oral Contraceptive Efficacy or Increase OC-Related Side Effects

Interacting Drug	Effect
Co-trimoxazole	Increases ethinyl estradiol blood levels; norgestrel unaffected (data sparse)
Fluconazole	Increases EE blood levels; data convincing

Source: Adapted from Goldzieher JW, 1998 (see reference 3).

Table 19

Drugs Whose Activity May Be Modified by Oral Contraceptive Use

Interacting Drug	Documentation	Management
Analgesics Acetaminophen	Adequate	Larger doses of analgesic may be required
Aspirin	Probable	Larger doses of analgesic may be required
Meperidine	Suspected	Smaller doses of analgesic may be required
Morphine	Probable	Larger doses of analgesic may be required
Anticoagulants (dicumarol, warfarin)	Controversial	
Antidepressants Imipramine	Suspected	Decrease dosage by about one-third
Other tricyclics	No data	

Tranquilizers
Diazepam,
  Alprazolam,
  Nitrazepam
	Suspected	Decrease dose

Temazepam	Possible	May need to increase dose
Other benzodiazepines	Suspected	Observe for increased effect
Anti-inflammatories (corticosteroids)	Adequate	Watch for potentiation of effects, decrease dose accordingly

Bronchodilators
(aminophylline,
  theophylline,
  caffeine)
	Adequate	Reduce starting dose by one-third

Antihypertensives Cyclopenthiazide, guanethidine	Adequate	Increase dose
Metoprolol	Suspected	May need to lower dose
Antibiotics Troleandomycin	Suspected liver damage	Avoid
Cyclosporine	Possible	May use smaller dose

Source: Adapted from Goldzieher JW, 1998 (see reference 3).

Table 20

Drugs That May Reduce Oral Contraceptive Efficacy

Interacting Drug	Documentation
Antituberculosis (rifampin)	Established
Antifungals (griseofulvin)	Strongly suspected
Anticonvulsants and Sedatives (phenytoin, ethotoin, mephenytoin, phenobarbital, primidone, carbamazepine, ethosuximide)	Strongly suspected; clinical trials data lacking
Antibiotics Tetracycline, doxycycline	Two small studies find no association
Penicillins	No association documented
Ciprofloxacin	No effect on efficacy of a 30 μg EE plus desogestrel OC
Ofloxacin	No effect on efficacy of a 30 μg EE plus levonorgestrel OC
Temafloxacin	No evidence of escape ovulation

Source: Adapted from Goldzieher JW, 1998 (see reference 3).

Take Home Messages

- *Strong evidence suggests griseofulvin, rifampin, and anticonvulsants that induce hepatic enzymes decrease the effect of OCs*

- *No sound evidence suggests that other antibiotics decrease the efficacy of OCs*

- *Other drugs that interact with OCs include certain analgesics, anti-inflammatories (corticosteroids), bronchodilators, and antihypertensives*

Anticonvulsants that increase OC metabolism

- *Epileptic women choosing to use combination OCs may need a higher-dose OC if they use medications that induce hepatic enzymes*

Continued on next page

Take Home Messages *(continued)*

- *Pharmacokinetic data suggest using an OC containing a progestin with minimal first-pass metabolism in order to achieve the greatest bioavailability and maintain adequate contraceptive protection*

- *The exact dosage is impossible to predict, due to individual variations in metabolism*

Antibiotics

- *Extra precautions (eg, a latex condom) are probably not warranted, but have been suggested*

Griseofulvin or rifampin

- *If the patient chooses OCs, increase the OC dosage or recommend condoms for dual protection*

References

1. Mattson RH, Cramer JA, Darney PD, et al. Use of oral contraceptives by women with epilepsy. *JAMA* 1986;256:238-240.

2. Back DJ, Orme MLE. Pharmacokinetic drug interactions with oral contraceptives. *Clin Pharmacokinet* 1990;18:472-484.

3. Goldzieher JW. *Hormonal Contraception: Pills, Injections & Implants*. 4th ed. Ontario: EMIS-CANADA; 1998:52-57.

4. Fraser IS, Jansen RPS. Why do inadvertent pregnancies occur in oral contraceptive users? Effectiveness of oral contraceptive regimens and interfering factors. *Contraception* 1983;27:531-551.

5. Weaver K, Glasier A. Interaction between broad-spectrum antibiotics and the combined oral contraceptive pill. A literature review. *Contraception* 1999;59:71-78.

6. Back DJ, Breckenridge AM, Challiner M, et al. The effect of antibiotics on the enterohepatic circulation of ethinylestradiol and norethisterone in the rat. *J Steroid Biochem* 1978;9:527-531.

7. Back DJ, Breckenridge AM, MacIver M, et al. The effects of ampicillin on oral contraceptive steroids in women. *Br J Clin Pharmacol* 1982;14:43-48.

8. Friedman CI, Huneke AL, Kim MH, et al. The effect of ampicillin on oral contraceptive effectiveness. *Obstet Gynecol* 1980;55:33-37.

9. De Groot AC, Eshuis H, Stricker BHC. Oral contraceptives and antibiotics in acne. *Br J Dermatol* 1991;124:212.

10. Hughes BR, Cunliffe WJ. Interactions between the oral contraceptive pill and antibiotics. *Br J Dermatol* 1990;122:717-718.

11. Joshi JV, Joshi VM, Sankholi GM, et al. A study of interaction of low-dose combination oral contraceptive with ampicillin and metronidazole. *Contraception* 1980;22:643-652.

12. Murphy AA, Zacur HA, Charache P, et al. The effect of tetracycline on levels of oral contraceptives. *Am J Obstet Gynecol* 1991;164:28-33.

13. Neely JL, Abate M, Swinker M, et al. The effect of doxycycline on serum levels of ethinyl estradiol, norethindrone, and endogenous progesterone. *Obstet Gynecol* 1991;77:416-420.

14. Van Dijke CPH, Weber JCP. Interaction between oral contraceptives and griseofulvin. *BMJ* 1984;288:1125-1126.

15. Scholten PC, Droppert RM, Zwinkels MGJ, et al. No interaction between ciprofloxacin and an oral contraceptive. *Antimicrob Agents Chemother* 1998; 42:3266-3268.

16. Csemiczky G, Alvendal C, Landgren BM. Risk for ovulation in women taking a low-dose oral contraceptive (Microgynon) when receiving antibacterial treatment with a fluoroquinolone (ofloxacin). *Adv Contracept* 1996;12: 101-109.

17. Back DJ, Tija J, Martin C, et al. The lack of interaction between temafloxacin and combined oral contraceptive steroids. *Contraception* 1991;43:317-323.

3.1: Health Benefits

Oral contraceptives provide substantial health benefits. In addition to their protective effect against ovarian and endometrial cancers, OCs provide well-documented protection against benign breast disease, ectopic pregnancy, dysmenorrhea, iron deficiency anemia, and salpingitis requiring hospitalization. Growing evidence also suggests that OCs may slow or prevent loss of bone mineral density in the premenopausal years and potentially protect against colorectal cancer. Protective effects against other conditions—uterine fibroids, toxic shock syndrome, and rheumatoid arthritis—also have been suggested. Pending the outcomes of further studies, however, these latter findings remain unproven.

Importantly, however, evidence concerning health benefits comes from studies of high-dose OCs. Almost no evidence exists concerning the effect of low-dose OCs (≤35 μg estrogen) on such health benefits as ovarian and endometrial cancers and benign breast disease. How lowering the doses of both estrogen and progestin will impact noncontraceptive health benefits is unknown.

Well-Established Noncontraceptive Benefits
Ovarian Cancer

Users of oral contraceptives are less likely to develop ovarian cancer than never users.[1,2] The biological mechanism of protection from ovarian cancer afforded by OCs is thought to involve avoidance of incessant ovulation or suppression or reduction of pituitary gonadotropin levels. The largest investigation to date, the Cancer and Steroid Hormone (CASH) Study, found an average 40% decrease in the future likelihood of ovarian cancer in women who had ever taken OCs.[2] A protective effect has been observed with as little as 3 to 6 months of OC use, with further declines in risk accompanying longer periods of use. For example, use for 7 years or more confers about a 60% to 80% reduction in risk.[1]

In addition, the effect persists for at least 15 years after the oral contraceptives are stopped. The finding that the reduction of ovarian cancer risk persists 15 years after last OC use is important in view of the increased incidence of this disease in older women. Risks of each of the four main histologic subtypes of epithelial ovarian cancer—serous, mucinous, endometrioid, and clear cell—are similarly reduced. The CASH investigators also found no difference in the amount of protection afforded by different OC formulations.[2]

Evidence also suggests that OCs can provide primary prevention for women at high risk of ovarian cancer.[3] A case-control study of 207 women with hereditary ovarian cancer and 161 of their sisters (who served as controls) found significant protection against ovarian cancer with high-dose OC use.[3] The high-risk women had the BRCA1 or BRCA2 genetic mutation, which confers a high lifetime risk of ovarian cancer. The adjusted odds ratio for ovarian cancer associated with any past use of oral contraceptives compared with no use was 0.5 (95% CI, 0.3-0.8). The protection was greatest, 70% reduction in risk, with 6 or more years of use (RR=0.3; 95% CI, 0.1-0.7).

Furthermore, data from England and Wales suggest that OCs already have reduced the age-specific incidence of and mortality from ovarian cancer.[4] Age-adjusted ovarian cancer mortality rates for all women increased steadily from 1950 to 1970 and then leveled off. When data were divided into older and younger age groups, however, mortality increased among women over 55 years of age, but decreased 26% among those ages 25 to 54 years (who were most likely to have used OCs) (Figure 22).

OCs appear to be responsible for the observed decline in ovarian cancer mortality. Among the cohort of women born between 1930 and 1934, death rates fell; 50% had exposure to the pill and 30% already took the pill by the age of 29 years. According to the authors, several facts support the assumption that the widespread use of oral contraceptives may be responsible for the decline in ovarian cancer mortality. One, "the incidence has not increased in the younger women, whereas it is certainly doing so among women over 55. ...[In addition] there is a consistent decrease in ovarian cancer mortality experienced by successive birth cohorts since 1936, and ...this trend is compatible with patterns of use of oral contraceptives [despite a trend for decreasing parity, which would tend to increase the risk of ovarian cancer]."[4]

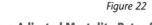

Figure 22

Age-Adjusted Mortality Rates for Ovarian Cancer in England and Wales

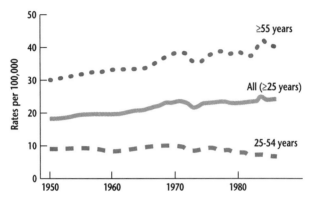

Source: Villard-Mackintosh L, et al, 1989 (see reference 4).

Endometrial Cancer

Although ovarian cancer is responsible for more deaths than other gynecologic cancers, endometrial cancer is the most common gynecologic cancer affecting American women.[5] With combination OC use for 12 months or longer, researchers have found a reduced risk of each of three major histological subtypes of endometrial cancer—adenocarcinoma, adenoacanthoma, and adenosquamous carcinoma.[6]

The risk of endometrial cancer is about 50% lower overall in pill users than in never users (Figure 23).[7] The reduced risk depends upon duration of use. Estimates suggest that risk is reduced by 20% with 1 year of use, 40% with 2 years of use, and 60% with 4 or more years of use.[1] The CASH Study found declines in risk with extended duration of OC use and a persistent risk reduction for at least 15 years after discontinuation.[6] The lasting nature of the protective effect is important because most endometrial cancers occur in women over 50 years of age.

The mechanism of the effect of OCs on the endometrium presumably is mediated by progestin. Researchers hypothesize that

Figure 23

Selected Case-Control Studies of Oral Contraception and Endometrial Cancer

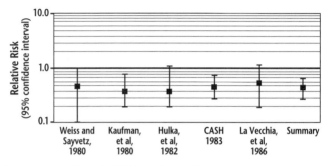

Source: Prentice RL, et al, 1987 (see reference 7).

endometrial cells may be less susceptible to carcinogenic changes after OC use. Not all studies agree as to whether different formulations provide equal protection against endometrial cancer.[1,6] One study suggests that formulations containing greater amounts of progestin may provide greater protection.[8]

Data from England and Wales also suggest that endometrial cancer mortality and incidence are declining.[9] These declines are occurring despite an upswing in related factors that increase the incidence of the disease. Risk factors include those increasing exposure to unopposed estrogen—low parity, late age at first full-term birth, young age at menarche, and late menopause. Vital statistics show a decrease for endometrial cancer mortality (41%) and morbidity (15%) in women under 55 years of age, suggesting an important protective effect of OCs on this disease.[9]

Benign Breast Disease

A reduced incidence of benign breast disease—including both fibrocystic changes and fibroadenomas—is among the most consistently demonstrated benefits of OC use.[10-13] The pill's favorable effects on benign breast disease have been attributed to inhibition of breast cell proliferation normally occurring in the first half of an ovulatory menstrual cycle.

Two prospective studies from the United Kingdom found risk reduction to be greater with formulations containing larger amounts of progestin.[14,15] One of these, the Oxford Family Planning Association (FPA) Study, also found decreasing risk of benign breast disease (both fibroadenomas and chronic cysts) with increasing years of OC use.[15] Studies note significant decreases in fibrocystic changes beginning after 1 to 2 years of OC use.[13] Current users appear to be at lowest risk of developing benign breast disease, with protection persisting for at least 1 year following pill discontinuation. A reduced risk of benign breast disease is evident across all age groups.

Pelvic Inflammatory Disease

OCs offer important protection against hospitalization for salpingitis or pelvic inflammatory disease (PID). Several mechanisms may contribute to the protective effect of OCs against PID. Thickening of the cervical mucus caused by the progestin could impede the ascent of pathogens into the endometrial cavity or enhance immunological factors. This is consistent with the reduction in PID risk also found with long-acting progestin methods. Decreased menstrual flow also may be a factor.

Oral contraceptive use is associated with a protective effect against hospitalization for PID (Figure 24).[16-18] One large, multicenter, case-control study evaluated 648 women hospitalized with an initial episode of PID and 2,516 hospitalized control subjects. The relative risk of PID for women using OCs was 0.5 (95% CI, 0.4-0.6).[16]

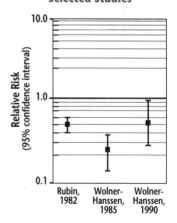

Figure 24

Relative Risk of Hospitalization for Acute Pelvic Inflammatory Disease among OC Users vs Contraceptive Nonusers: Selected Studies

Sources: Adapted from references 16-18.

Two other large, case-control studies also reported significant reductions in PID risk among OC users. A study of 738 women reported a 76% reduction in risk of acute salpingitis in OC users vs nonusers (RR=0.2; 95% CI, 0.1-0.4).[17] Another case-control study examined 141 women with verified PID (by laparoscopy and/or endometrial biopsy) and 739 randomly selected, sexually active controls. Researchers reported a 50% reduction in PID risk among OC users vs nonusers (RR=0.5; 95% CI, 0.3-0.9).[18]

The studies only include women who were hospitalized with the diagnosis of PID. Because the majority of women with PID are treated on an outpatient basis, the studies are not necessarily generalizable to all PID patients. Thus, the current medical literature cannot determine whether a protective effect exists for ambulatory cases of PID.

Ectopic Pregnancy

By inhibiting ovulation, OCs protect against ectopic pregnancy and associated mortality and morbidity. Case-control studies demonstrate 90% protection from ectopic pregnancy with current OC use.[7,11] The risk of ectopic pregnancy among OC users is about 0.005 ectopic pregnancies per 1,000 woman-years of use.[19]

Functional Ovarian Cysts

Older epidemiologic studies found the risk of developing functional ovarian cysts decreased with the use of OCs.[7,11,20] Newer data suggest, however, that this effect is attenuated by the lower steroid dosage in currently used pills. In a population-based, case-control study, Holt et al assessed the effect of current use of monophasic or triphasic OCs on the risk of functional ovarian cyst development.[21] Cases were all 15- to 39-year-old enrollees in the Group Health Cooperative of Puget Sound who had a primary diagnosis of functional ovarian cyst. Compared with women not using hormonal contraception, women currently using OCs had a relative risk of a diagnosed functional ovarian cyst of 0.8 (95% CI, 0.4-1.8) for users of monophasic OCs. Users of triphasic OCs had a relative risk of 1.3 (95% CI, 0.5-3.3) (Figure 25).

A cohort study identified almost 7,500 women, aged 15 to 44 years, enrolled in Maine Medicaid who were prescribed OCs.[22] Thirty-two women had a principal diagnosis of functional ovarian

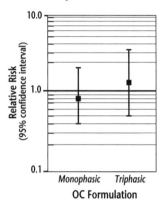

Figure 25

Relative Risk of a Diagnosed Ovarian Cyst among Current Users, by OC Formulation

Source: Holt VL, et al, 1992 (see reference 21).

cyst confirmed by medical records as being >20 mm in diameter. Compared to women not using OCs, women using OCs had a nonsignificant lower incidence of cysts. The effect was greatest among users of higher-dose estrogen pills (OR=0.2; 95% CI, 0.01-1.3) and lower for users of low-dose monophasic pills with ≤35 µg estrogen (OR=0.5; 95% CI, 0.2-1.3). Researchers found the least protection for multiphasic pills (OR=0.9; 95% CI, 0.3-2.3).

Menstrual Cycle Benefits

Fewer menstrual disorders —eg, heavy, irregular menstruation or intermenstrual bleeding—occur in OC users than in women having spontaneous menstrual cycles.[13] OC use also improves primary dysmenorrhea in most women and premenstrual tension in some. This effect may particularly benefit teenage patients, among whom dysmenorrhea is a common complaint. Perimenopausal women can also benefit from regular menstrual cycles during a time of increasingly irregular cycles due to hormonal fluctuations. While these conditions seldom pose any serious threat to health, they frequently impair quality of life.

Iron Deficiency Anemia

Combination OCs lessen menstrual blood loss, which reduces the likelihood of iron deficiency anemia. Both current and past OC use have been associated with a protective effect.[11]

Growing Evidence
Bone Density

Growing evidence suggests that OCs may preserve bone mineral density, which normally starts to decline between the ages of 30 and 40 years. Since 1991, several studies of both college-aged and postmenopausal women provide support for this health benefit.[23-25] A cross-sectional, retrospective study by Kleerekoper et al investigated risk factors for low bone mineral density in a group of almost 2,300 women, 76% of whom were postmenopausal.[23] Thirty percent of the women in the study reported prior OC use. The investigators found that a history of OC use was protective against low bone mineral density (OR=0.4; 95% CI, 0.2-0.5).

Further analyses demonstrated an increasing protective effect with increasing duration of use. Women who reported using OCs for 10 years or longer gained the greatest protection (OR=0.2; 95% CI, 0.1-0.7) when compared with women who had never used OCs (Figure 26). These results held true whether the measurements were taken from the distal radius and ulna or lumbar spine; however, effects on the femoral head (and potential for hip fracture) were not evaluated. Because the mean age of the study participants was high (54 years), it is likely that most OC users took higher-dose pills. More work needs to be done to examine the effect of low-dose OCs on postmenopausal bone density.

Figure 26

Risk of Low Bone Density by Duration of OC Use

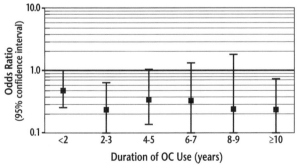

Source: Kleerekoper M, et al, 1991 (see reference 23).

A 1996 review of the literature weighed the evidence for and against OCs protecting against bone loss.[26] Overall, the weight of the evidence suggests that premenopausal use of OCs is beneficial for preserving bone mass; eight studies supported an association while four did not. How much estrogen is optimal is unknown. Although OCs may help to preserve bone density, neither the Royal College of General Practitioners nor the Oxford FPA have found protection against various types of fractures in primarily pre-menopausal OC users.[27,28]

On the other hand, a population-based, case-control study of postmenopausal women in Sweden found a protective effect of OC use against hip fracture.[29] The questionnaire survey of women in largely urban areas of Sweden interviewed 1,327 cases and 3,312 controls. Ever use of any OCs provided a significantly lower risk of hip fracture (OR=0.8; 95% CI, 0.6-0.9). Ever use of high-dose OCs (≥50 μg estrogen) conferred a 40% reduction in risk (OR=0.6; 95% CI, 0.4-0.8). Age during use of OCs was important. Women who used OCs at 40 years of age and older had significant protection against hip fracture (any OC use, OR=0.7; 95% CI, 0.5-0.9), while OC users under age 30 years and those 30 to 39 years had smaller, but nonsignificant, reductions in risk of hip fracture.

Colorectal Cancer

Some evidence suggests that OCs may protect women against the later development of colorectal cancer. In North America and Europe, incidence and mortality of large bowel cancer have been consistently lower among women than among men. One possible explanation involves exposure to endogenous or exogenous sex hormones.

One recent investigation found a 40% reduction in risk among women who had ever used OCs (OR=0.6; 95% CI, 0.4-0.9).[30] Use for 2 or more years conferred a 50% reduction in risk (OR=0.5; 95% CI, 0.3-1.0). Although several studies have found a similar protection with OC use,[31,32] others have not.[33-35] Also, the relationship between duration of use and reduction of risk has been inconsistent; therefore, caution is warranted in interpretation of these findings.

The most recent analysis of the Nurses' Health Study found some evidence of a protective effect of OCs against colorectal

Figure 27

**Relative Risk of Colorectal Cancer by Duration of OC Use
— Nurses' Health Study**

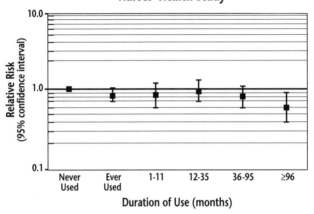

Source: Martinez ME, et al, 1997 (see reference 36).

cancer.[36] This large, prospective cohort study found a trend of increasing protection with longer duration of use (Figure 27). The data included 12 years of follow-up (over 1 million person-years) from 1980 through 1992. The investigators identified 501 cases of colorectal cancer. Women using OCs for 96 months or longer had a relative risk of 0.6 (95% CI, 0.4-0.9; p for trend=0.02). Whether these results apply to women taking current low-dose pills remains unknown, however, as most women in the cohort had likely taken high-dose OC preparations.

Limited Evidence
Uterine Leiomyomas

The Oxford Family Planning Association researchers noted a reduced risk of uterine leiomyomas (fibroids) in OC users.[37] Increasing protection correlated with a longer duration of pill use; 10 years of use conferred a 30% risk reduction. A large, case-control study from Italy also found a significantly reduced risk of fibroids with 7 or more years of OC use compared to no use (OR=0.5; 95% CI, 0.3-0.9)[38]; an earlier report, however, found no effect.[39] Importantly, the use of OCs in women with fibroids does not worsen this condition and may help diminish bleeding.[40]

Toxic Shock Syndrome

Toxic shock syndrome (TSS) has been associated with use of tampons during menstruation and with higher tampon absorbency. Five studies of TSS reported an overall 50% reduction in risk associated with OC use.[41] However, two subsequent, large, case-control studies—one of menstrual TSS and the other of non-menstrual TSS—failed to demonstrate such an effect.[42,43] The latter findings may be explained by subsequent changes in tampon composition, absorbency, and usage. Because of decreased menstrual bleeding, OC users may have been less likely to use highly absorbent tampons than were other women. Other factors not examined may have played a role, as well.

Rheumatoid Arthritis

Two studies conducted before 1982 demonstrated a 40% to 50% reduction in the risk of premenopausal rheumatoid arthritis in OC users.[44,45] Since that time, 12 studies—eight case-control and four cohort—have yielded conflicting results. Biases in these observational studies subsequently have been identified, however, which complicate attempts to correlate OC use and risk of rheumatoid arthritis. A meta-analysis of all studies published through 1996 found no conclusive evidence of a protective effect of OCs; additional work is needed before any firm conclusions can be drawn.[46]

Take Home Messages

- *OCs have many noncontraceptive health benefits, including protection against the following:*

Well Documented

Life-Threatening Diseases

- Ovarian cancer
- Pelvic inflammatory disease requiring hospitalization
- Endometrial cancer
- Ectopic pregnancy

Continued on next page

Take Home Messages *(continued)*

Diseases Affecting Quality of Life
- Benign breast disease
- Dysmenorrhea
- Iron deficiency anemia

Growing Evidence
- Low bone density
- Colorectal cancer

Limited Evidence
- Uterine fibroids
- Toxic shock syndrome
- Rheumatoid arthritis

References

1. Schlesselman JJ. Cancer of the breast and reproductive tract in relation to use of oral contraceptives. *Contraception* 1989;40:1-38.

2. The Cancer and Steroid Hormone Study of the Centers for Disease Control and the National Institute of Child Health and Human Development. The reduction in risk of ovarian cancer associated with oral contraceptive use. *N Engl J Med* 1987;316:650-655.

3. Narod SA, Risch H, Moslehi R, et al. Oral contraceptives and the risk of hereditary ovarian cancer. *N Engl J Med* 1998;339:424-428.

4. Villard-Mackintosh L, Vessey MP, Jones L. The effects of oral contraceptives and parity on ovarian cancer trends in women under 55 years of age. *Br J Obstet Gynaecol* 1989;96:783-788.

5. American Cancer Society. *Cancer Facts and Figures-1996*. Atlanta: American Cancer Society; 1996.

6. The Cancer and Steroid Hormone Study of the Centers for Disease Control and the National Institute of Child Health and Human Development. Combination oral contraceptive use and the risk of endometrial cancer. *JAMA* 1987;257:796-800.

7. Prentice RL, Thomas DB. On the epidemiology of oral contraceptives and disease. *Adv Cancer Res* 1987;49:285-401.

8. Rosenblatt KA, Thomas DB, the WHO Collaborative Study of Neoplasia and Steroid Contraceptives. Hormonal content of combined oral contraceptives in relation to the reduced risk of endometrial carcinoma. *Int J Cancer* 1991; 49:870-874.

9. Villard-Mackintosh L, Murphy M. Endometrial cancer trends in England and Wales: a possible protective effect of oral contraception. *Int J Epidemiol* 1990; 19:255-258.

10. Mishell DR Jr. Noncontraceptive benefits of oral contraceptives. *J Reprod Med* 1993;38:1021-1029.

11. Peterson HB, Lee NC. The health effects of oral contraceptives: misperceptions, controversies, and continuing good news. *Clin Obstet Gynecol* 1989;32:339-355.

12. Ory HW. The noncontraceptive health benefits from oral contraceptive use. *Fam Plann Perspect* 1982;14:182-184.

13. Mishell DR. Noncontraceptive health benefits of oral steroidal contraceptives. *Am J Obstet Gynecol* 1982;142:809-816.

14. Royal College of General Practitioners' Oral Contraception Study. Effect on hypertension and benign breast disease of progestagen component in combined oral contraceptives. *Lancet* 1977;1:624.

15. Brinton LA, Vessey MP, Flavel R, et al. Risk factors for benign breast disease. *Am J Epidemiol* 1981;113:203-214.

16. Rubin GL, Ory HW, Layde PM. Oral contraceptives and pelvic inflammatory disease. *Am J Obstet Gynecol* 1982;144:630-635.

17. Wolner-Hanssen P, Svensson L, Mardh P, et al. Laparoscopic findings and contraceptive use in women with signs and symptoms suggestive of acute salpingitis. *Obstet Gynecol* 1985;66:233-238.

18. Wolner-Hanssen P, Eschenbach DA, Paavonen J, et al. Decreased risk of symptomatic chlamydial pelvic inflammatory disease associated with oral contraceptive use. *JAMA* 1990;263:54-59.

19. Franks AL, Beral V, Cates W Jr, et al. Contraception and ectopic pregnancy risk. *Am J Obstet Gynecol* 1990;163:1120-1123.

20. Vessey M, Metcalfe A, Wells C, et al. Ovarian neoplasms, functional ovarian cysts, and oral contraceptives. *BMJ* 1987;294:1518-1520.

21. Holt VL, Daling JR, McKnight B, et al. Functional ovarian cysts in relation to the use of monophasic and triphasic oral contraceptives. *Obstet Gynecol* 1992;79:529-533.

22. Lanes SF, Birmann B, Walker AM, et al. Oral contraceptive type and functional ovarian cysts. *Am J Obstet Gynecol* 1992;166:956-961.

23. Kleerekoper M, Brienza RS, Schultz LR, et al. Oral contraceptive use may protect against low bone mass. *Arch Intern Med* 1991;151:1971-1976.

24. Recker RR, Davies M, Hinders SM, et al. Bone gain in young adult women. *JAMA* 1992;268:2403-2408.

25. Kritz-Silverstein D, Barrett-Connor E. Bone mineral density in postmenopausal women as determined by prior oral contraceptive use. *Am J Public Health* 1993;83:100-102.

26. DeCherney A. Bone-sparing properties of oral contraceptives. *Am J Obstet Gynecol* 1996;174:15-20.

27. Cooper C, Hannaford P, Croft P, et al. Oral contraceptive pill use and fractures in women: a prospective study. *Bone* 1993;14:41-45.

28. Vessey M, Mant J, Painter R. Oral contraception and other factors in relation to hospital referral for fracture. Findings in a large cohort study. *Contraception* 1998;57:231-235.

29. Michaëlsson K, Baron JA, Farahmand BY, et al. Oral contraceptive use and risk of hip fracture: a case-control study. *Lancet* 1999;353:1481-1484.

30. Fernandez E, La Vecchia C, D'Avanzo B, et al. Oral contraceptives, hormone replacement therapy and the risk of colorectal cancer. *Br J Cancer* 1996;73:1431-1435.

31. Potter JD, McMichael AJ. Large bowel cancer in women in relation to reproductive and hormonal factors: a case-control study. *J Natl Cancer Inst* 1983;71:703-709.

32. Furner SE, Davis FG, Nelson RL, et al. A case-control study of large bowel cancer and hormone exposure in women. *Cancer Res* 1989;49:4936-4940.

33. Kune GA, Kune S, Watson LF. Oral contraceptive use does not protect against large bowel cancer. *Contraception* 1990;41:19-25.

34. Weiss NS, Daling JR, Chow WH. Incidence of cancer of the large bowel in women in relation to reproductive and hormonal factors. *J Natl Cancer Inst* 1981;67:57-60.

35. Bostick RM, Potter JD, Kushi LH, et al. Sugar, meat, fat intake, and non-dietary risk factors for colon cancer incidence in Iowa women (United States). *Cancer Causes Control* 1994;5:38-52.

36. Martinez ME, Grodstein F, Giovannucci E, et al. A prospective study of reproductive factors, oral contraceptive use, and risk of colorectal cancer. *Cancer Epidemiol Biomark Prev* 1997;6:1-5.

37. Ross RK, Pike MC, Vessey MP, et al. Risk factors for uterine fibroids: reduced risk associated with oral contraceptives. *BMJ* 1986;293:359-362.

38. Chiaffarino F, Parazzini F, La Vecchia C, et al. Use of oral contraceptives and uterine fibroids: results from a case-control study. *Br J Obstet Gynaecol* 1999;106:857-860.

39. Parazzini F, Negri E, LaVecchia C, et al. Oral contraceptive use and risk of uterine fibroids. *Obstet Gynecol* 1992;79:430-433.

40. Friedman AJ, Thomas PP. Does low-dose combination oral contraceptive use affect uterine size or menstrual flow in premenopausal women with leiomyomas? *Obstet Gynecol* 1995;85:631-635.

41. Gray RH. Toxic shock syndrome and oral contraception. *Am J Obstet Gynecol* 1987;156:1038.

42. Schwartz B, Gaventa S, Broome CV, et al. Nonmenstrual toxic shock syndrome associated with barrier contraceptives: report of a case-control study. *Rev Infect Dis* 1989;11(suppl):S43-S48.

43. Reingold AL, Broome CV, Gaventa S, et al. Risk factors for menstrual toxic shock syndrome: results of a multi-state case-control study. *Rev Infect Dis* 1989;11(suppl):S35-S41.

44. Wingrave SJ. Reduction in incidence of rheumatoid arthritis associated with oral contraceptives: Royal College of General Practitioners' Oral Contraception Study. *Lancet* 1978;1:569-571.

45. Vandenbroucke JP, Boersma JW, Festen JJM, et al. Oral contraceptives and rheumatoid arthritis: further evidence for a preventive effect. *Lancet* 1982;2:839-842.

46. Pladevall-Vila M, Delclos GL, Varas C, et al. Controversy of oral contraceptives and risk of rheumatoid arthritis: meta-analysis of conflicting studies and review of conflicting meta-analyses with special emphasis on analysis of heterogeneity. *Am J Epidemiol* 1996;144:1-14.

3.2: Treatment of Medical Disorders

The use of oral contraceptives to treat medical problems is often related to the well-documented health benefits that the pill provides. OCs can treat dysmenorrhea, abnormal uterine bleeding, bleeding disorders, polycystic ovary syndrome, acne, and hirsutism. Clinicians sometimes also use OCs to replace estrogen in amenorrheic patients and alleviate conditions affected by the menstrual cycle, such as endometriosis, mood swings, and menstrual migraine.

Prescribing a drug for indications other than those approved by the FDA is both legal and common. Indeed, practitioners often prescribe medications for unlabeled uses without being aware that the indication is not approved. Acknowledging that some clinicians may be reluctant to prescribe "off-label," the FDA has clearly stated that they may prescribe drugs for unapproved uses.

The American Medical Association (AMA) echoes the FDA's position on unlabeled use of medications. According to the AMA, the "prescription of a drug for an unlabeled indication is entirely proper if based on rational scientific theory, reliable medical opinion, or controlled clinical studies. The FDA has made eminently clear that it neither has nor wants the authority to compel prescribers to adhere to officially labeled uses. ....Drug labeling *per se* does not set the standard for what is good medical practice."[1] Ironically, many health insurers cover OCs as a benefit for off-label uses, such as dysmenorrhea, irregular cycles, or endometriosis, but not the labeled use of contraception.

Menstrual Disorders

One of the most common off-label uses of oral contraceptives is for relief of menstrual disorders. OC users have fewer instances of menorrhagia (excessive uterine bleeding), irregular menstruation, and intermenstrual bleeding than women experiencing spontaneous menstrual cycles.[2,3]

Dysmenorrhea

OC use improves primary dysmenorrhea in most women.[3-5] The usefulness of OCs in treating dysmenorrhea may be particularly beneficial for adolescents. Dysmenorrhea is a common complaint among teenagers; as many as 60% of adolescents report the condition, 14% of whom have missed school as a result.[6] The alleviation of dysmenorrhea also may enhance compliance. OC users who experience the beneficial effect on dysmenorrhea may be more likely to take their pills regularly.[7]

OCs should not be considered first-line therapy for dysmenorrhea in nonsexually active teens. The primary treatment for dysmenorrhea is nonsteroidal anti-inflammatory drugs. If that treatment is insufficient, then OCs are a reasonable option, unless contraindications are present.

Excessive or Unpatterned Uterine Bleeding

Abnormal uterine bleeding, commonly referred to as dysfunctional uterine bleeding (DUB), is defined as excessive, prolonged, unpatterned uterine bleeding in the absence of an identifiable pathologic condition.[8] Menorrhagia is quite common, affecting about 20% of reproductive age women.[9] The problem is particularly prevalent among adolescents, in whom abnormal bleeding is often related to anovulatory cycles resulting from an immature hypothalamic-pituitary-ovarian axis.

OCs are used to treat heavy and intermenstrual bleeding, restore synchrony to the endometrium, and prevent long-term consequences of anovulation.[8] Inhibiting the synthesis of estrogen receptors with synthetic progestin can reduce endometrial activity and regulate menstrual blood loss.[1] However, progestin alone may not stop the bleeding if the condition has been prolonged; in that case, combined estrogen-progestin OCs are preferred.

A recent Cochrane Collaboration review found sufficient evidence to support the benefits of OCs for heavy menstrual bleeding: "A range of medical therapies is prescribed in order to reduce excessive menstrual blood loss, including prostaglandin synthetase inhibitors, antifibrinolytics, the oral contraceptive pill [OCP] and other hormones. Objective data have shown that, at least in the short term, considerable reduction in the volume of menses is achievable. ...When taken in a cyclical fashion, [the OC pill] induces regular shedding of a thinner endometrium and inhibits ovulation. With this method, good cycle control can be achieved and, together with the provision of contraception, this makes OCP a most acceptable longer term therapy for some women with menorrhagia."[10]

Citing insufficient data from randomized controlled trials, however, the Cochrane reviewers were unable to quantify the effectiveness of oral contraceptives as treatment for irregular, heavy, or intermenstrual bleeding. Other reviews have reported that OCs may reduce menstrual flow by up to 53%.[8]

The recommended OC treatment regimen depends upon bleeding severity. For acute episodes, especially with anemia, a high-dose estrogen-progestin approach suppresses bleeding.[11] Up to three or four OC tablets a day can be used. Once the bleeding stops, high-dose therapy is stopped, or tapered and stopped, to allow withdrawal bleeding. After the acute bleeding episode is controlled, the patient can use a standard-dose OC regimen if she desires. For less acute episodes without anemia, regimens of one or two OCs a day are usually successful.

Bleeding Disorders

A small percentage of women with heavy menstrual bleeding may have bleeding disorders. Leukemia, idiopathic thrombocytopenia, and von Willebrand's disease need to be ruled out, particularly in adolescents.

Oral contraceptives may be beneficial in treating bleeding disorders, particularly von Willebrand's disease, because combination OCs are associated with an increase in von Willebrand's factor.[11] Other patients who can benefit from OCs include women taking anticoagulants who are at risk of intraperitoneal hemorrhage from ovulation.

Polycystic Ovary Syndrome

OCs have been used to treat conditions related to excess androgens, such as polycystic ovary syndrome (PCOS). The characteristics of PCOS include a history of chronic anovulatory bleeding combined with clinical and laboratory evidence of androgen excess, such as elevated serum androgen concentrations, acne, and hirsutism. PCOS is also associated with infertility, insulin resistance, and obesity. Because women with PCOS often have chronic estrogen exposure unopposed by progesterone, they have an increased risk for endometrial cancer, as well.[12] They also are at increased risk for the development of diabetes mellitus.

PCOS is one of the most common reproductive endocrinological disorders in women.[12] A recent study of 369 reproductive age women reported a PCOS prevalence of 4% and a hirsutism prevalence of 7% (Figure 28).[13] PCOS was defined as oligo-ovulation, clinical hyperandrogenism and/or hyperandrogenemia, and exclusion of other related disorders, such as hyperprolactinemia, thyroid abnormalities, and nonclassical adrenal hyperplasia. Hirsutism was defined by a Ferriman-Gallwey body hair quantification score of 6 or more. The study reported a slightly higher percentage of PCOS and hirsutism among white women than among black women; however, the difference was not statistically significant.[13]

The primary goal of PCOS treatment is to alleviate symptoms. The risk of sequelae also may be reduced by treatment. The most frequently used approaches are ovulation induction for infertility, OCs or a progestin for menstrual irregularity, and OCs and/or spironolactone for hirsutism.[12,14] OCs also can be effective in treating PCOS-induced acne.[15] (For further discussion of how combination OCs affect adrenal androgen production, see the section

Figure 28

Prevalence of Hirsutism and Polycystic Ovary Syndrome (PCOS) in US Women by Race

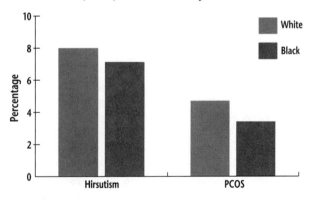

Source: Knochenhauer ES, et al, 1998 (see reference 13).

on androgenicity.) Insulin sensitizing agents (eg, metformin) also have been studied to reduce androgens, induce ovulation, and as adjunctive therapy for those with type 2 diabetes mellitus.

Acne and Hirsutism

OCs can treat acne and hirsutism in women with and without PCOS. Combination OCs suppress ovarian, adrenal, and peripheral androgen metabolism, resulting in a net reduction in free testosterone. In addition, OCs inhibit 5α-reductase in the skin, resulting in lower levels of the active androgen dihydrotestosterone.

Numerous studies have reported acne improvement with various OC formulations (Table 21).[16-23] However, data are scant with regard to comparisons among and between various formulations. No randomized controlled trials have found that one preparation is better treatment for existing acne than others.

Table 21

Acne Improvement in Women Using Combination OCs with Various Progestins: Results of Selected Studies

Study	Progestin(s)	Results
Palatsi, et al, 1984[16]	levonorgestrel, desogestrel	Serum free testosterone fell 60% in both groups; significant improvement in acne
Lemay, et al, 1990[17]	levonorgestrel	Acne improved in 69% of patients
Louden, et al, 1990[18]	levonorgestrel, gestodene	Both groups had a similar improvement in acne
Wishart, 1991[19]	levonorgestrel, cyproterone acetate	Both groups had a 72% reduction in acne counts
Weber-Diehl, et al, 1992[20]	gestodene	50% reduction in incidence of acne
Redmond, et al, 1997[21]	norgestimate vs placebo	46% reduction in total lesions
Lucky, et al, 1997[22]	norgestimate vs placebo	53% decrease in total lesion count
Thorneycroft, et al, 1999[23]	levonorgestrel, norethindrone acetate	Both groups had a similar improvement in acne

Sources: See references 16-23.

One OC has been approved by the FDA for the treatment of acne in women over 15 years of age who desire contraception and are unresponsive to topical antiacne medications. Two randomized placebo-controlled trials found significant improvement in preexisting acne among users of this triphasic OC, which contains 35 µg EE and norgestimate.[21,22] The trials did not compare this pill to any other OCs.

OCs are not first-line treatment for acne, however. Topical therapies are the first choice, followed by oral antibiotics. If moderate or severe acne remains, OCs can be used as the next step. OCs should be considered before or concurrently with isotretinoin (Accutane®), given that this acne medication is teratogenic.

Endometriosis

Endometriosis, which may affect up to 15% of premenopausal women, can cause pelvic pain, dysmenorrhea, dyspareunia, and infertility.[24] Endometriosis most likely results from an abnormal immunologic response to retrograde menstruation with resultant implantation of endometrial tissue in the pelvis. Consequently, OCs and other birth control methods that alter menstrual flow may influence the development of endometriosis.

Clinicians sometimes use OCs to help reduce the pelvic pain associated with endometriosis and for long-term suppression after initial surgical or medical treatment. For example, many clinicians use OCs as maintenance after treatment for 3 to 6 months with a gonadotropin-releasing hormone analogue. One approach, the tricycle regimen, consists of taking three cycles of OCs without a break for withdrawal bleeding. This regimen reduces menses to four occasions per year, thus reducing the number of opportunities for retrograde menstruation and additional endometrial tissue deposits, and results in less frequent dysmenorrhea.

A recent Cochrane Collaboration review examined the evidence related to OC use for endometrial pain.[24] According to the reviewers, "There is a paucity of data relating to the use of oral contraceptive preparations in the treatment of symptomatic endometriosis. [However,] the data, such as it is, supports the common practice of the use of the oral contraceptive pill as first-line therapy. ...It may offer an acceptable long-term alternative treatment for the painful symptoms of endometriosis."[24]

Ovarian Cysts

Although some clinicians prescribe OCs to hasten the regression of existing ovarian cysts, little evidence supports this action. The original, uncontrolled case-series report by Spanos described the use of 6 weeks of high-dose OC therapy to hasten regression of functional ovarian cysts in order to make a differential diagnosis between cysts and ovarian neoplasms easier.[25] A 1990 randomized controlled trial of the effect of OC therapy on adnexal cysts in women of reproductive age, however, found no benefit. Forty-eight patients with cysts were randomized to receive either 1 mg norethindrone/50 μg mestranol per day or no treatment for up to 6 weeks.[26] At 6 weeks, the cysts had resolved in all but one patient in each group. By 9 weeks, both groups had complete resolution of their cystic adnexal masses.

Two possible explanations may account for the lack of benefit observed. The lack of benefit may be due to low power of the study (a small sample size) or to the use of an inadequate dose of steroids to suppress the cysts. Also, the majority of women had cysts that were hormonally induced; therefore, the findings may not be applicable to spontaneously ovulating women. A similar, but larger, study of women with spontaneously occurring cysts will be required to settle this issue.

Diet- or Exercise-Induced Amenorrhea

OCs have been prescribed for estrogen replacement in patients with hypoestrogenic amenorrhea. This condition is common among women with eating disorders and those who are involved in activities such as running or ballet. Many clinicians prescribe OCs for these young women, as observational studies have suggested a benefit of hormone replacement.[27-29] The best therapy, however, is for these women to gain weight, particularly if they have eating disorders, so they have spontaneous resumption of menses. Young women with severe eating disorders who become hypoestrogenic early in adolescence may not recover bone density even if they regain their weight and menses later. Most studies of the effect of estrogen replacement on bone density have been done with postmenopausal women, however. The applicability of these studies to amenorrheic adolescents is not clear.[30]

OCs also may benefit other amenorrheic patients, such as young women who have had bilateral oophorectomy or radiation therapy for cancer. Oral contraceptives can be given to these patients as a primary way of replacing estrogen.

Menstrual Cycle-Related Conditions

OCs may help a number of conditions that are linked to the menstrual cycle, including mood changes and menstrual migraines. The sharp variations in serum estradiol and progesterone levels during the menstrual cycle can trigger these conditions. By contrast, women using monophasic OCs have relatively constant hormonal levels throughout most of the cycle.

OCs may be helpful in managing menstrual mood disorders. Randomized controlled trials show benefits of OCs for premenstrual syndrome (PMS) in some situations; in other cases, they do not.[31] Advantages of OCs for PMS include low cost and reversibility.

OCs also may be useful in treating other conditions that are exacerbated by menses, such as menstrual migraines.[32] Menstrual migraines can sometimes be managed by longer cycles of OCs— using 42 or 63 days of active pills, rather than 21 days. Women with a history of headache relief while on OCs or those with intractable menstrual migraine may be the most appropriate candidates for OC therapy.[33] (For further discussion, see the section on headache/migraine.)

Take Home Messages

■ *OCs can be used to treat a variety of medical disorders, including:*

- *Dysmenorrhea*
- *Excessive or unpatterned uterine bleeding*
- *Endometriosis*
- *Polycystic ovary syndrome*
- *Bleeding disorders (eg, von Willebrand's disease)*
- *Acne*
- *Hirsutism*
- *Menstrual cycle-related conditions (menstrual migraine, premenstrual syndrome)*
- *Diet- or exercise-induced amenorrhea*

References

1. American Medical Association. Prescription practices and regulatory agencies. In: *Drug Evaluations,* 6th ed. Philadelphia: W.B. Saunders; 1986:1-11.

2. Crosignani PG, Vegetti W, Bianchedi D. Hormonal contraception and ovarian pathology. *Eur J Contracept Reprod Health Care* 1997;2:207-211.

3. Mishell DR. Noncontraceptive health benefits of oral steroidal contraceptives. *Am J Obstet Gynecol* 1982;142:809-816.

4. Privrel T, Daubenfeld O. Clinical experience in Switzerland with the new monophasic oral contraceptive Minulet (75 µg gestodene, 30 µg ethinyl oestradiol). *Br J Clin Pract* 1988;42:292-298.

5. Ulstein M, Svendsen E, Steier A, et al. Clinical experience with a triphasic oral contraceptive. *Acta Obstet Gynecol Scand* 1984;63:233-236.

6. Klein JR, Litt IF. Epidemiology of adolescent dysmenorrhea. *Pediatrics* 1981; 68:661-664.

7. Robinson JC, Plichta S, Weisman CS, et al. Dysmenorrhea and use of oral contraceptives in adolescent women attending a family planning clinic. *Am J Obstet Gynecol* 1992;166:578-583.

8. Lavin C. Dysfunctional uterine bleeding in adolescents. *Curr Opin Pediatr* 1996;8:328-332.

9. Stabinsky SA, Einstein M, Breen JL. Modern treatments of menorrhagia attributable to dysfunctional uterine bleeding. *Obstet Gynecol Survey* 1998; 54:61-72.

10. Iyer V, Farquahr C, Jepson R. Oral contraceptive pills for heavy menstrual bleeding (Cochrane Review). In: *The Cochrane Library,* Issue 2, 1999. Oxford: Update Software.

11. Chuong CJ, Brenner PF. Management of abnormal uterine bleeding. *Am J Obstet Gynecol* 1996;175:787-792.

12. Guzick D. Polycystic ovary syndrome: symptomatology, pathophysiology, and epidemiology. *Am J Obstet Gynecol* 1998;179:S89-S93.

13. Knochenhauer ES, Key TJ, Kahsar-Miller M, et al. Prevalence of the polycystic ovary syndrome in unselected black and white women of the southeastern United States: a prospective study. *J Clin Endocrinol Metab* 1998;83:3078-3082.

14. American College of Obstetricians and Gynecologists. Evaluation and treatment of hirsute women. *ACOG Technical Bulletin* 1995;203.

15. Berga SL. The obstetrician-gynecologist's role in the practical management of polycystic ovary syndrome. *Am J Obstet Gynecol* 1998;179:S109-S113.

16. Palatsi R, Hirvensalo E, Liukko P, et al. Serum total and unbound testosterone and sex hormone binding globulin (SHBG) in female acne patients treated with two different oral contraceptives. *Acta Derm Venereol* 1984;64:517-523.

17. Lemay A, Dewailly SD, Grenier R, et al. Attenuation of mild hyperandrogenic activity in postpubertal acne by a triphasic oral contraceptive containing low doses of ethinyl estradiol and d,l-norgestrel. *J Clin Endocrinol Metab* 1990;71:8-14.

18. Loudon NB, Kirkman RJE, Dewsbury JA. Double-blind comparison of Femodene and Microgynon. Eur J Obstet Gynecol Reprod Biol 1990;34: 257-266.

19. Wishart JM. An open study of Triphasil and Diane 50 in the treatment of acne. *Australas J Dermatol* 1991;32:51-54.

20. Weber-Diehl F, Unger R, Lachnit-Fixson U. Triphasic combination of ethinyl estradiol and gestodene. *Contraception* 1992;46:19-27.

21. Redmond GP, Olson WH, Lippman JS, et al. Norgestimate and ethinyl estradiol in the treatment of acne vulgaris: a randomized, placebo-controlled trial. *Obstet Gynecol* 1997;89:615-622.

22. Lucky AW, Henderson TA, Olson WH, et al. Effectiveness of norgestimate and ethinyl estradiol in treating moderate acne vulgaris. *J Am Acad Dermatol* 1997;37:746-754.

23. Thorneycroft IH, Stanczyk FZ, Bradshaw KD, et al. Effect of low-dose oral contraceptives on androgenic markers and acne. *Contraception* 1999;60:255-262.

24. Moore J, Kennedy S, Prentice A. Modern combined oral contraceptives for pain associated with endometriosis (Cochrane Review). In: *The Cochrane Library,* Issue 2, 1999. Oxford: Update Software.

25. Spanos WJ. Preoperative hormonal therapy of cystic adnexal masses. *Am J Obstet Gynecol* 1973;116:551-556.

26. Steinkampf MP, Hammond KR, Blackwell RE. Hormonal treatment of functional ovarian cysts: a randomized, prospective study. *Fertil Steril* 1990;54:775-777.

27. Cumming DC. Exercise-associated amenorrhea, low bone density, and estrogen replacement therapy. *Arch Intern Med* 1996;156:2193-2195.

28. Chen EC, Brzyski RG. Exercise and reproductive dysfunction. *Fertil Steril* 1999;71:1-6.

29. Warren MP, Stiehl AL. Exercise and female adolescents: effects on the reproductive and skeletal systems. *J Am Med Womens Assoc* 1999;54:115-120,138.

30. Hergenroeder AC. Bone mineralization, hypothalamic amenorrhea, and sex steroid therapy in female adolescents and young adults. *J Pediatr* 1995;126:683-689.

31. Daugherty JE. Treatment strategies for premenstrual syndrome. *Am Fam Physician* 1998;58:183-192.

32. Sulak PJ, Cressman BE, Waldrop E, et al. Extending the duration of active oral contraceptive pills to manage hormone withdrawal symptoms. *Obstet Gynecol* 1997;89:179-183.

33. Silberstein SD, Merriam GR. Sex hormones and headache. *J Pain Symptom Manage* 1993;8:98-114.

3.3: Media, OCs, and Patient Fears

Unbalanced or inaccurate media coverage in newspapers, magazines, and television has created public perceptions of the birth control pill that are unwarranted. Although some misperceptions have declined in recent years, women continue to overestimate health risks of oral contraceptives and are largely unaware of the pill's noncontraceptive health benefits.

Negative media reporting contributes to OC discontinuation and patient misperceptions. An in-depth analysis of use of OCs and the IUD between 1970 and 1975 documented increased rates of stopping OCs after unfavorable news stories about the methods appeared in print and on television.[1] Rates of discontinuation climbed for 5 to 6 months after negative publicity. Other surveys have revealed a tendency to overreport risks of OCs, particularly breast cancer, and underreport health benefits.[2,3] The most recent pill scare occurred in 1995, when the UK's drug regulatory agency warned patients about venous thromboembolism risks with OCs containing desogestrel or gestodene. The warning scared women and caused an increase in unintended pregnancy and abortion.[4-8]

In early 1994, ACOG announced the results of a Gallup poll on US women's attitudes toward contraception, a long-awaited update to a similar 1985 survey.[9,10] While the study showed a decline in the percentage of women who believed there were substantial health risks associated with OC use (76% to 54%), the proportion who cited cancer as the chief risk remained constant at approximately 30% (Figure 29). Only 6% of respondents were aware of the potential protective effect against cancer and 42% said OCs provided no health benefits other than prevention of pregnancy.[9]

A similar 1993 study of women coming to the Yale University Health Services' Department of Obstetrics and Gynecology (students, faculty, and employees) produced comparable results, suggesting that educational status has little effect on misperceptions about OCs (Figure 30).[11] In this study, 49% of women believed there were substantial risks to using the pill—close to half (47%) thought OCs caused breast cancer. Furthermore, between 80% and 95% of respondents were unaware of health benefits asso-

Figure 29

Comparison of Selected Results from the ACOG/Gallup Poll on Attitudes toward Contraception, 1985 and 1994

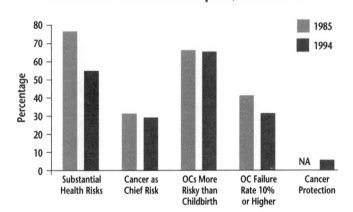

Sources: American College of Obstetricians and Gynecologists, 1985 and 1994 (see references 9 and 10).

Figure 30

Risks of Oral Contraceptives Cited by Women Faculty, Students, and Employees of Yale University*

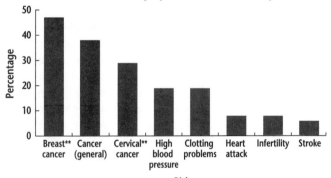

* Response to an open-ended question
** Response to a specific, multiple-choice question

Source: Peipert JF, et al, 1993 (see reference 11).

Figure 31

Sources of Contraceptive Information

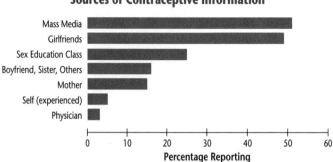

Source: Herold ES, et al, 1980 (see reference 12).

ciated with OC use. The findings indicate that patients seeking OCs are likely to harbor myths, fears, and misperceptions about the method.

A Canadian study of adolescent women found that 51% stated they had received most of their information concerning OCs from the media—as opposed to only 3% receiving OC information from a physician (Figure 31).[12] The Canadian study also found that mothers were the source of contraceptive information for 15% of the adolescents. The mothers of many teenagers today are familiar with OCs that were available in the 1960s and 1970s—pills that were high-dose and caused more nuisance side effects, such as nausea. During the 1970s, the media often highlighted negative stories about the pill (eg, the Nelson congressional pill hearings in 1970). Thus, mothers of today's teens may be giving their daughters obsolete information about oral contraceptives.

Misperceptions about oral contraceptives also exist in developing countries.[13] Family Health International conducted a survey of women of reproductive age in Thailand, Sri Lanka, Egypt, Senegal, Nigeria, Mexico, Costa Rica, and Chile. About 50% to 75% of the women believed OCs carry substantial health risks. Among the non-African women, over 40% thought that taking the pill is more dangerous than childbearing. Similar to the ACOG and Yale reports, the researchers also found that the health benefits of OCs were virtually unknown.

Take Home Messages

- *Negative media messages about OCs have influenced perceptions and use of this method both in the United States and developing countries*

- *Many women believe OCs carry substantial health risks*

- *Few women (<20%) are aware of the health benefits of OCs*

References

1. Jones EF, Beniger JR, Westoff CF. Pill and IUD discontinuation in the United States, 1970-1975: the influence of the media. *Fam Plann Perspect* 1980;12: 293-300.

2. Grimes DA. Breast cancer, the pill and the press. In: Mann RD, ed. *Oral Contraceptives and Breast Cancer*. Pearl River, New York: Parthenon Publishing Group, Inc.; 1989:309-318.

3. Lebow MA. The pill and the press: reporting risk. *Obstet Gynecol* 1999;93: 453-456.

4. Wood R, Botting B, Dunnell K. Trends in conceptions before and after the 1995 pill scare. *Popul Trends* 1997;89:5-12.

5. Armstrong JL, Reid M, Bigrigg A. Scare over oral contraceptives. Effect on behavior of women attending a family planning clinic. *BMJ* 1995;311:1637. Letter.

6. Ramsey S. UK "pill scare" led to abortion increase. *Lancet* 1996;347:1109.

7. Seamark CJ. Scare over oral contraceptives. Effect on women in a general practice in Devon... *BMJ* 1995;311:1637. Letter.

8. Furedi A, Paintin D. Conceptions and terminations after the 1995 warning about oral contraceptives. *Lancet* 1998;352:323-324.

9. The Gallup Organization. *Attitudes Toward Contraception*. A poll conducted for the American College of Obstetricians and Gynecologists. Princeton, NJ: March 1985.

10. American College of Obstetricians and Gynecologists. *Poll shows women still skeptical of contraceptive safety (press release)*. Washington, DC: ACOG; January 20, 1994.

11. Peipert JF, Gutmann J. Oral contraceptive risk assessment: a survey of 247 educated women. *Obstet Gynecol* 1993;82:112-117.

12. Herold ES, Goodwin MS. Perceived side effects of oral contraceptives among adolescent girls. *Can Med Assoc J* 1980;123:1022-1026.

13. Grubb GS. Women's perceptions of the safety of the pill: a survey in eight developing countries. *J Biosoc Sci* 1987;19:313-321.

3.4: Successful OC Use

Oral contraceptives have a failure rate of approximately 7% during the first 12 months of typical use.[1] Failure rates among certain subgroups, such as adolescents or women of lower socioeconomic status, are even higher.[2] The main reason for contraceptive failure among OC users is improper pill taking, including inconsistent use, missed pills, and incorrect transition between pill packs. A related concern that contributes to unintended pregnancy is discontinuation due to problems or concerns related to the method, which occurs among one-third of all OC users during the first 12 months of use.[3]

Incorrect pill taking and OC discontinuation often result from fear, misunderstanding, and forgetfulness. Patients may misunderstand pill instructions, be uncertain as to how to cope with missed pills, or have unfounded fears or misunderstandings about side effects. Common mistakes include incorrect transition between pill packs, running out of pills, or skipping tablets (Table 22). Studies of how women take the pill have found that many use it incorrectly (Table 23).[4-7] The 1995 National Survey of Family Growth (NSFG) found that only 71% of women reported taking one pill every day. Among teens 15 to 19 years of age, 28% missed two or more OC pills during the 3 months prior to the interview.[8]

According to an analysis of the 1995 NSFG, 16% of women who used the pill indicated that they missed two or more pills during the prior 3 months. Inconsistent OC use was twice as common among Hispanic and non-Hispanic black women than among white women and those of other ethnic groups. In addition, OC users who recently began use (within the past 3 to 6

Table 22

Examples of Inconsistent OC Use

- Not filling or refilling the OC prescription
- Forgetting to take pills
- Running out of pills
- Starting the next pack late
- Taking pills incorrectly
- Using sporadically
- Not using a backup method when needed

Table 23

Pill Taking: Selected Study Results

- Only 28% of patients took the pill correctly.[4]

- Only 42% took a pill every day.[5]

- 16% had pills left at the end of the month.[5]

- Approximately 33% of adolescents missed a pill in the previous 3 months.[6]

- 17% did not know they needed a 7-day break with 21-day pill packs.[7]

months) were almost three times more likely than longer-term users to report inconsistent use.[9] Another factor associated with inconsistency of pill use was having had an unintended pregnancy.

Addressing Fears

Several studies have documented exaggerated fears and misperceptions about OCs among women.[10-12] Among adolescents, fear of weight gain is particularly widespread—86% of teens seen in a suburban practice setting reported the concern.[10] Other researchers have found that teens who perceived substantial health-related problems with the pill were least likely to continue to use it.[13] More than half of all OC users believe the pill carries substantial health risks.[11] Chief among these are fear of breast cancer and cervical cancer. Fear of high blood pressure and clotting problems also are prevalent.[12]

Table 24

Helpful Initial Steps in OC Counseling

1. Uncover fears

- *What does the woman believe about the pill?*
  eg, women often fear OCs cause cancer and weight gain

- *Misperceptions*
  eg, body needs a "rest"

2. Provide facts

- *No overall increased risk of cancer*

- *OCs have many health benefits*
  eg, menstrual cycle regulation and alleviation of dysmenorrhea

Patient counseling to counteract exaggerated perceptions of OC risks can be helpful, particularly with new users. Clinicians need to uncover patient fears about the pill as an initial step. No matter what other counseling steps are taken, if the patient has unexpressed reservations about taking the pill, she may eventually stop taking it without informing her health care provider (Table 24). By addressing patient fears, clinicians create an opportunity to encourage consistent pill use. Often, these fears are not something that clinicians would expect. Ask patients what they have heard and be sensitive to their fears and concerns.

Clinicians can ask, "What do you know about oral contraceptives? Have you ever taken the pill before? What was your experience? Do you think the pill has any benefits?" These questions allow a patient to generate her own responses before the clinician addresses the issues (Figure 32). These questions should be asked both before the patient goes on the pill and again during the first follow-up visit.

A thorough approach to counseling may help improve method satisfaction. A recent nationwide, prospective cohort study of 943 OC users reported that the perceived quality of the patient-provider relationship correlated with OC satisfaction. Women who reported high satisfaction with the counseling they received were also the most satisfied OC users, even after controlling for other factors that predicted method satisfaction (RR=2.2; 95% CI, 1.4-3.5).[14]

Figure 32

Effective Patient Counseling Includes Uncovering and Addressing Fears about the Pill

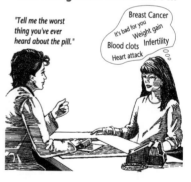

Anticipating Side Effects

In addition to addressing initial patient concerns, clinicians should prepare new OC users for any side effects they may experience. In fact, possible side effects may require considerable discussion to prevent discontinuation. Even the *perception* of side effects can lead to noncompliance. Breakthrough bleeding, amenorrhea, actual or perceived weight gain, nausea, headaches, and perceived mood changes are among the usually transient side effects that can affect OC compliance (Figure 33). Clinicians should educate patients about these nuisance side effects, clarify any misperceptions, and provide advice on how to manage side effects.

Figure 33

Side Effects and Inconsistent Use: "Minor" Side Effects May Lead to Major Consequences

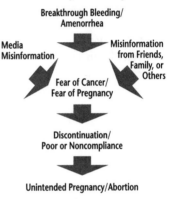

Clear Pill-Use Instructions

New OC users need to understand clearly how to take their oral contraceptives (eg, first day vs Sunday start). One step in patient counseling is to be sure the patient knows how to take her OCs correctly. This includes showing the patient the pill package and the order in which to take the pills (Figure 34). Clinicians should reinforce the key message: *Take one pill every day—at the same time every day.* Scheduling follow-up visits within 1 to 2 months is another strategy that can improve compliance with OCs.

Clinicians should help the patient link pill taking with some other regular daily activity, such as brushing her teeth. Other potentially effective measures include setting an alarm on a pager or cellular phone. Having a regular pill-taking routine helps ensure consistent OC use—women who lack an established routine are 3.6 times more likely to miss two or more pills per cycle than those who have a regular routine (RR=3.6; 95% CI, 2.1-6.3).[14]

Clear verbal instructions are particularly important with adolescent OC users. Some teens accidentally lose their written pill instructions; others may dispose of the instructions because they

Figure 34

Three Things to Tell a New OC User

1. *When to Start:* Sunday or first day of menses
ACTION: Show patient the pill package

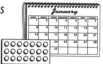

 2. *Take One Pill Every Day*
ACTION: Establish a time of day to take pill and
cue to a daily activity; eg, brushing teeth

3. *Minor Side Effects:* Breakthrough bleeding/nausea are
common and transitory — they will likely go away
ACTION: Give patient the clinic/contact person phone number
and advise her to call with any concerns

do not want them to be found at home. For this reason, both
written and verbal instructions are helpful. One approach is to go
over written instructions with teens and conduct a question-and-
answer session before they leave the office to help them commit
the instructions to memory.

OC users need to understand what to do if they miss pills
because missing tablets is common.[8,14] In general, clinicians should
instruct patients to take a missed pill as soon as they remember. If
patients miss two or more pills in a row, instructions vary; however,
generally, women should take the forgotten pills and use a backup
method of birth control for the next 7 days. Practitioners should
review this information with patients and encourage them to
call the office or clinic if they have any questions. (For further discussion of what to do in case of missed pills, see the section on
starting OCs.)

When patients do call with questions or concerns about oral
contraceptive use, listening to the problem and providing reassurance, when appropriate, are important. Listening to the patient is
an essential first step. Phone calls may provide an ideal opportunity
for further education and reinforcement; for example, if a woman
calls about an episode of breakthrough bleeding, the clinician can
ask whether she has been taking her pills at the same time every
day and suggest a strategy that will help her do so.

Stressing Health Benefits

Clinicians may want to discuss noncontraceptive OC benefits with new users (Table 25). This information may help encourage correct and consistent use of the method and improve satisfaction. For example, a patient who breaks up with her boyfriend may stop taking the pill because she does not anticipate having sexual intercourse in the next few weeks or months. Women who understand that OCs have substantial health benefits, however, may continue to take the pill even if they perceive themselves as not needing it for contraception. In a recent study, women who were aware of no more than one beneficial effect of OC use were more than twice as likely to be dissatisfied than those who knew of four or more benefits (RR=2.2; 95% CI, 1.3-3.6).[14] (For additional suggestions to enhance successful OC use, see Table 26.)

Counseling about menstrual cycle benefits may help improve satisfaction. Many women find cycle regularity, lighter periods, and relief of dysmenorrhea welcome effects of the pill. This is especially true for teenagers and for women over age 40, who are more likely to experience cycle irregularity and increased menstrual flow. Relief of dysmenorrhea, in particular, is one health benefit that may help adolescents (and adult women) continue to take their pills successfully.[15] Use of combined OCs in the older age group also helps avoid the onset of menopausal symptoms and aids in the transition to postmenopausal hormone replacement therapy.

Table 25

OC Health Benefits to Emphasize

Teens	*Women over 35 years*
• Cycle regularity	• Protection against endometrial and ovarian cancers
• Relief of dysmenorrhea	
• Acne improvement	• Preservation of bone density
• No net weight gain	• Regular cycles and consistent hormonal levels up to menopause
• Protection against hospitalization for pelvic inflammatory disease	• Improvement in fibrocystic breast changes

Table 26

Additional Suggestions for Enhancing Successful OC Use

- Include an additional cycle in the refill prescription, if possible, to accommodate missed pills or lost packets.

- Discuss the use of a backup method and the availability of emergency contraception.

- Discuss prevention of sexually transmitted diseases. Provide a condom and information about proper use.

- On follow-up visits, ask patients if they have had any problems taking their pills.

Take Home Messages

- *Women often fear the side effects of OCs*
- *Clinicians can help patients by dispelling fears, counseling about common side effects, and providing clear instructions on how to use the particular package of OCs*
- *Knowledge of health benefits may help women use OCs consistently*
- *Clinicians should pay special attention to counseling women who have recently begun OC use and those who have already experienced an unintended pregnancy*

References

1. Fu H, Darroch JE, Haas T, et al. Contraceptive failure rates: new estimates from the 1995 National Survey of Family Growth. *Fam Plann Perspect* 1999;31:58-63.

2. Hillard PJA. Oral contraception noncompliance: the extent of the problem. *Adv Contracept* 1992;8(suppl 1):13-20.

3. Trussell J, Vaughan B. Contraceptive failure, method-related discontinuation, and resumption of use: results from the 1995 National Survey of Family Growth. *Fam Plann Perspect* 1999;31:64-72,93.

4. Finlay IG, Scott MGB. Patterns of contraceptive pill taking in an inner city practice. *BMJ* 1986;293:601-602.

5. Oakley D, Parent J. A scale to measure microbehaviors of oral contraceptive pill use. *Social Biology* 1990;37:215-222.

6. Goldstuck ND, Hammar E, Butchart A. Use and misuse of oral contraceptives by adolescents attending a free-standing clinic. *Adv Contracept* 1987;3: 335-339.

7. Brook SJ. Do combined oral contraceptive users know how to take their pill correctly? *Br J Fam Plann* 1991;17:18-20.

8. Abma JC, Chandra A, Mosher WD, et al. Fertility, family planning, and women's health: new data from the 1995 National Survey of Family Growth. National Center for Health Statistics. *Vital Health Stat* 1997;23.

9. Peterson LS, Oakley D, Potter LS, et al. Women's efforts to prevent pregnancy: consistency of oral contraceptive use. *Fam Plann Perspect* 1998;30:19-23.

10. Emans SJ, Grace E, Woods ER, et al. Adolescents' compliance with the use of oral contraceptives. *JAMA* 1987;257:3377-3381.

11. American College of Obstetricians and Gynecologists. Poll shows women still skeptical of contraceptive safety (press release). January 20, 1994.

12. Peipert JF, Gutmann J. Oral contraceptive risk assessment: a survey of 247 educated women. *Obstet Gynecol* 1993;82:112-117.

13. Balassone ML. Risk of contraceptive discontinuation among adolescents. *J Adolesc Health Care* 1989;10:527-533.

14. Rosenberg MJ, Waugh MS, Burnhill MS. Compliance, counseling and satisfaction with oral contraceptives: a prospective evaluation. *Fam Plann Perspect* 1998;30:89-92,104.

15. Robinson JC, Plichta S, Weisman CS, et al. Dysmenorrhea and use of oral contraceptives in adolescent women attending a family planning clinic. *Am J Obstet Gynecol* 1992;166:578-583.

3.5: Myths

i. Weight Gain

In the United States, women are bombarded with messages from the mass media concerning the ideal body image. The ideal image is most often portrayed as slender, and women of all ages are subjected to the pressures of conforming. Under these circumstances, clinicians need to be aware that many women, particularly adolescents, fear weight gain as a consequence of using oral contraceptives.

No net weight gain occurs among women using OCs over 1 year compared to women using nonhormonal methods.[1,2] In fact, a randomized controlled trial done in the 1970s, when high-dose OCs were used, found no net weight gain among OC users.[3] At least one study has shown that suburban adolescents are highly concerned about weight gain and that even the *perception* of weight gain is enough to cause poor compliance.[4] Clinicians need to counsel patients carefully about this misperception. Patients should be weighed at each visit and be counseled about healthy eating habits and exercise. (For further discussion about weight gain, see the section on approach to common side effects of OCs.)

Take Home Messages

- *Many women, especially teenagers, fear OCs will make them gain weight*
- *Patients can be reassured that as many women lose as gain weight while taking OCs*
- *Patients should be weighed at each visit and counseled about healthy eating habits and exercise*

References

1. Carpenter S, Neinstein LS. Weight gain in adolescent and young adult oral contraceptive users. *J Adolesc Health Care* 1986;7:342-344.
2. Rosenberg M. Weight change with oral contraceptive use and during the menstrual cycle. Results of daily measurements. *Contraception* 1998;58:345-349.

3. Goldzieher JW, Moses LE, Averkin E, et al. A placebo-controlled double-blind crossover investigation of the side effects attributed to oral contraceptives. *Fertil Steril* 1971;22:609-623.

4. Emans SJ, Grace E, Woods ER, et al. Adolescents' compliance with the use of oral contraceptives. *JAMA* 1987;257:3377-3381.

ii. Taking a "Rest"

One of the myths that has surrounded the use of oral contraceptives is the idea that a woman should periodically take a "rest" from pill use. The origin of this myth has been attributed to a British family planning practitioner who wrote a letter to a prominent British medical journal suggesting that it would be a good idea for women to get off the pill once a year, although no scientific evidence was offered to support this suggestion.

No evidence suggests that taking a rest from the pill is medically necessary or beneficial. On the other hand, taking a rest from the pill may lead to negative consequences for the patient, such as unintended pregnancy and abortion. Studies have found that a woman who stops taking the pill may not use another form of birth control or may switch to a less effective method, thus increasing her risk of unintended pregnancy.[1,2]

In addition, taking a rest from the pill can perpetuate compliance problems. Such side effects as breakthrough bleeding, bloating, and nausea, which can initiate compliance problems, are common during the first few months of OC use. Discontinuing and restarting the pill may cause another few months of these unpleasant side effects, which are frequently perceived negatively by women and can result in compliance problems.

Given that no scientific evidence suggests a woman should take a rest from the pill, important advice for the patient is: "You do not need to take a 'rest' from the pill. Please call me first if you are thinking about stopping so we can discuss your concerns."

Take Home Messages

- *No evidence supports the common myth that women need to take a "rest" from the pill*
- *Taking a "rest" can lead to unintended pregnancy*

References

1.   Pratt WF, Bachrach CA. What do women use when they stop using the pill? *Fam Plann Perspect* 1987;19:257-266.

2.   Trussell J, Vaughn B. Contraceptive failure, method-related discontinuation, and resumption of use: results from the 1995 National Survey of Family Growth. *Fam Plann Perspect* 1999;31:64-72,93.

iii. Birth Defects

Many women are concerned about the possibility of birth defects with oral contraceptive use. For example, 11% of teens seen in an adolescent clinic were concerned that the pill would cause birth defects.[1] Two review articles and a recent meta-analysis found no association between oral contraceptives and teratogenic consequences.[2-4]

Some early reports suggested an association between OCs and such birth defects as anencephaly, transposition of the great vessels, limb reductions, and other gross malformations. A 1981 overview by Wilson and Brent, however, found that the use of exogenous hormones during pregnancy was not associated with abnormality in nongenital organs and tissues.[2]

The conclusions were based on several important findings. As the use of OCs increased, the incidence of the suspected birth defects would be expected to rise if a true association existed; however, surveillance data have shown that this is not the case. More reports in the literature show no association than suggest a relationship. No animal model has been able to demonstrate a causal relationship between administration of exogenous hormones in normal therapeutic doses, period of gestational development, and teratogenic effects. Furthermore, because hormones act specifically on target tissues, no reasonable biologic mechanism explains how exogenous sex hormones could act to damage nongenital fetal tissue.

A meta-analysis by Bracken calculated the relative risks of specific types of fetal malformations.[4] The relative risk from 12 prospective studies analyzed was 1.0 (95% CI, 0.8-1.2) for all malformations. Thus, no overall increased risk was found for birth defects. The specific relative risks for congenital heart and limb-reduction defects were 1.1 (95% CI, 0.7-1.6) and 1.0 (95% CI, 0.3-3.6), respectively. These data provide strong evidence that exposure to OCs in early pregnancy does not have a teratogenic effect. Furthermore, the progestin dosage of current OCs is so low that OCs pose no risk of causing masculinization of a female fetus. A woman who inadvertently takes OCs prior to or at the time of conception, or in early pregnancy, should be reassured that OCs do not cause birth defects.

Take Home Messages

- *OCs are not teratogenic*
- *Clinicians can reassure women that if inadvertent OC ingestion occurs during early pregnancy, it will not harm the fetus*

References

1. Emans SJ, Grace E, Woods ER, et al. Adolescents' compliance with the use of oral contraceptives. *JAMA* 1987;257:3377-3381.

2. Wilson JG, Brent RL. Are female sex hormones teratogenic? *Am J Obstet Gynecol* 1981;141:567-580.

3. Simpson JL, Phillips OP. Spermicides, hormonal contraception and congenital malformations. *Adv Contracept* 1990;6:141-167.

4. Bracken MB. Oral contraception and congenital malformations in offspring: a review and meta-analysis of the prospective studies. *Obstet Gynecol* 1990; 76:552-557.

iv. Post-Pill Amenorrhea

Little evidence exists to suggest that oral contraceptives cause "post-pill amenorrhea." Reports of post-pill amenorrhea, or irregular menstruation and anovulation, began appearing in the 1960s.[1,2] Estimates of its frequency ranged from 0.2% to 3%.[3] Researchers found that post-pill amenorrhea was more likely to occur in women who had never given birth and the condition was unrelated to duration of use.

Later reviews suggested that about half of post-pill amenorrhea cases were unrelated to OC use, and noted that OC use likely had masked an earlier condition. By 1981, estimates concerning post-pill amenorrhea indicated its occurrence to be less than one in 1,000.[4]

Because OCs are commonly used to treat menstrual cycle disorders, when OCs are discontinued, menstrual irregularity, including amenorrhea, often returns to its prior pattern.[5] Amenorrhea after discontinuation of OCs should be investigated to determine its cause; however, OC use likely masked the condition, rather than caused it.

Take Home Message

- *Amenorrhea that occurs after OC discontinuation (often called post-pill amenorrhea) most likely reflects a woman's menstrual pattern prior to OC use*

References

1. Shearman RP. Amenorrhea after treatment with oral contraceptives. *Lancet* 1966;2:1100-1101.

2. Whitelaw MJ, Nola VF, Kalman CF. Irregular menses, amenorrhea and infertility following synthetic progestational agents. *JAMA* 1966;195:780-782.

3. Rice-Wray E, Correu S, Gorodovsky J, et al. Return of ovulation after discontinuance of oral contraceptives. *Fertil Steril* 1967;18:212-218.

4. Hull MGR, Bromham DR, Savage PE, et al. Post-pill amenorrhea: a causal study. *Fertil Steril* 1981;36:472-476.

5. Goldzieher JW, Zamah NM. Oral contraceptive side effects: where's the beef? *Contraception* 1995;52:327-335.

v. Stunted Growth

Some young teens or their parents may be concerned about whether taking oral contraceptives will stunt a young woman's growth. The origin of this myth may stem from the known effect of estrogen on bone epiphyses. Young women predicted to have excessively tall stature are treated with high doses of estrogen for several years in order to accelerate bone maturation and limit final height. This practice may explain why an association has been suggested between OCs and incomplete growth.

Several factors make it unlikely that oral contraceptives could limit growth. Most young women are substantially past the age of menarche and maximal growth when OCs are prescribed. Skeletal maturation or "bone age" is often determined by comparing a radiograph of the wrist and hand with established standards. For example, a young woman found to have a bone age of 12.5 to 13 years (the typical age for menarche) has reached nearly 96% of final height. A young woman with a bone age of 14 years has reached 98% of her final height. Most importantly, current OCs have one-third to one-tenth the estrogen as the typical doses that are used daily (not in cycles) to treat tall stature.[1] Moreover, a German study of mestranol 80 µg given in cycles with progestin found a satisfactory reduction in predicted height only in adolescents with a bone age of 9 to 10 years.[2] Thus, current low-dose oral contraceptives given after menarche are highly unlikely to affect final height.

Take Home Messages

- *Most growth occurs prior to menarche*
- *OCs do not limit adolescent growth*

References

1. Prader A, Zachmann M. Treatment of excessively tall girls and boys with sex hormones. *Pediatrics* 1978;62(suppl):1202-1210.

2. Schambach H, Nitschke U. Treatment of constitutionally tall girls with physiological estrogen doses in the prepuberty period. An alternative to high-dose estrogen therapy. *Monatsschr-Kinderheilkd* 1985;133:32-37.

3.6: Discontinuing and Restarting

Contraceptive discontinuation contributes to the large number of unintended pregnancies in the United States.[1] Couples who discontinue an effective method, such as oral contraceptives, often increase their risk of unintended pregnancy by substituting a less effective means of contraception, such as condoms.

Of the 6 million pregnancies that occur each year in the US, about half (48%) are unintended (Figure 35). Half of those unintended pregnancies occur among couples who were actively practicing contraception; the remainder occur among couples who were not using a birth control method at the time of conception.[1] Women may stop using one method but fail to adopt any substitute method, placing them at high risk of unintended pregnancy. Of the roughly 1.5 million unintended pregnancies that occur annually among non-contracepting couples, many take place when couples discontinue a birth control method that they find inconvenient, difficult to use, or associated with unwanted side effects.[2]

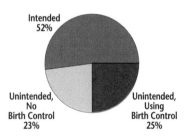

Figure 35

Percentage of Intended vs Unintended Pregnancies Annually in US by Birth Control Use

Intended 52%

Unintended, No Birth Control 23%

Unintended, Using Birth Control 25%

Source: Henshaw SK, 1998 (see reference 1).

1995 US Data

The 1995 National Survey of Family Growth (NSFG) examined discontinuation rates for various contraceptive methods and trends related to method resumption.[2] Overall, 31% of women discontinued use of a contraceptive for method-related reasons during the first 6 months of use. This number rose to 44% after 12 months of use (Figure 36). By 24 months, more than 60% discontinued their initial contraceptive for method-related reasons.[2]

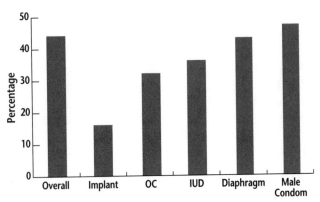

Figure 36

Percentage of Women Discontinuing Contraception During the First 12 Months of Use for Method-Related Reasons—1995 NSFG*

*National Survey of Family Growth

Source: Trussell J, et al, 1999 (see reference 2).

Oral contraceptives had the second lowest set of discontinuation rates following subdermal implants. After the first 6 months of use, about one in five OC users quit for method-related reasons. OC discontinuation rates rose steadily over time, reaching 32% after 12 months. Within 24 months of starting the method, roughly half of OC users had discontinued.[2]

In general, the likelihood of contraceptive discontinuation was associated with age and future childbearing intentions. When all reversible contraceptives were considered together, women aged 30 years or older were 28% less likely to discontinue than were younger women. Women who wanted to have a child in the future were 24% more likely to stop using contraception for method-related reasons than those who did not.[2]

Most women who discontinued a contraceptive method began using another method shortly thereafter. Within 1 month of discontinuing, 68% of women were again using contraception. This number increased to 76% after 3 months, 79% after 6 months, and 82% after 12 months.[2]

Factors associated with contraceptive resumption include age, parity, and income. According to the 1995 NSFG analysis, "Compared with women aged 20-29 [years], women younger than 20 are 7% more likely to resume use and those aged 30 or older are 14% less likely. Women with two or more children are 17% more likely to resume use than are primiparous or nulliparous women. The rate of resumption of use is 7% lower among low-income women and 8% higher among high-income women than among middle-income women."[2]

OC Discontinuation Factors

The 1995 NSFG also found that socioeconomic factors were associated with oral contraceptive discontinuation. Lower-income women (those with family incomes less than 150% of the federal poverty level) were 39% more likely to discontinue OCs than those with higher incomes.[2]

Side effects and OC discontinuation are related. A 1995 study analyzed a convenience sample of almost 6,700 current or former OC users aged 16 to 30 years from Denmark, France, Italy, Portugal, and the United Kingdom.[3] In each country, interviewers selected women on the street from several locations in two large cities. Logistic regression enabled investigators to determine the independent effect of factors influencing discontinuation. While reported findings reflect the women's stated reasons for discontinuation, they do not take into account other potential factors, such as an unstated desire to become pregnant.

The most common reason women gave for discontinuing OCs was side effects. Roughly 51% of women reported at least one side effect. OC discontinuation during the first 2 years of use occurred almost twice as frequently in women reporting nausea, breast tenderness, and bleeding irregularities in the first 3 months compared to women not reporting the same side effects.[3]

Two estrogen-related side effects—nausea and breast tenderness—were among those most strongly associated with OC discontinuation (Figure 37). Women experiencing nausea were twice as likely to discontinue OCs than those users not experiencing the side effect (RR=2.1; 95% CI, 1.7-2.7). Those experiencing

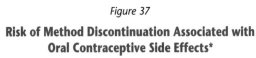

Figure 37

Risk of Method Discontinuation Associated with Oral Contraceptive Side Effects*

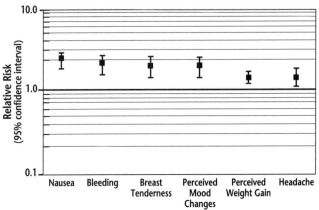

*Versus women not reporting the side effect (referent group)

Source: Rosenberg MJ, et al, 1995 (see reference 3).

breast tenderness (RR=1.8; 95% CI, 1.4-2.3) were 80% more likely to discontinue OCs.[3] Women reporting perceived mood changes (RR=1.8; 95% CI, 1.4-2.2) also had a high risk of discontinuation.

The risk of OC discontinuation increased with the number of side effects a woman experienced (Figure 38). On average, a woman experiencing one OC side effect was 1.5 times more likely to stop using the method compared with a user who did not experience side effects (RR=1.5; 95% CI, 1.3-1.8). OC users who experienced two different side effects were more than twice as likely to discontinue (RR=2.2; 95% CI, 1.8-2.8); those with three side effects were more than three times as likely to quit (RR=3.2; 95% CI, 2.4-4.4).[3] All of these risks applied to a general population of OC users; they were not related to any specific formulation.

Implications for Clinicians

Another survey found that more than four-fifths of OC discontinuers either failed to adopt a subsequent method or adopted one

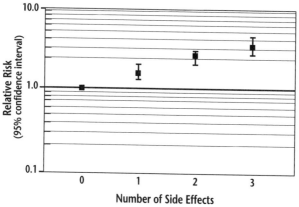

Figure 38

Risk of OC Discontinuation among Users Experiencing Multiple Side Effects

Source: Rosenberg MJ, et al, 1995 (see reference 3).

Figure 39

Contraceptive Methods Used by Women within 3 Months of OC Discontinuation

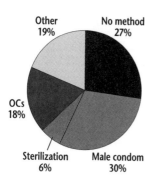

Source: Trussell J, et al, 1999 (see reference 2).

that was less effective.[4] In addition, the 1995 NSFG found that more than a quarter (27%) of OC discontinuers were using no method of birth control 3 months after stopping OCs (Figure 39). Thirty percent were using male condoms, 6% chose sterilization, and 19% opted for other methods of contraception. The remaining 18% had resumed oral contraceptive use within 3 months of stopping OCs.[2]

Most women stopping OCs place themselves at increased risk of unintended pregnancy. In many cases, discontinuation is the result of "nuisance" side

201

effects that are transient in nature. By providing anticipatory counseling, especially for new OC users, clinicians can help patients expect minor side effects and understand their transitory nature. Some women have a higher risk for OC discontinuation and may need special counseling and follow-up.

Take Home Messages

- In the 1995 NSFG, among women experiencing unintended pregnancy, half were using birth control
- Low-income women are 30% to 40% more likely to discontinue OCs
- Side effects, particularly nausea, bleeding, breast tenderness, and mood changes, significantly increase discontinuation of OCs
- Among OC discontinuers, about 20% resume OCs within 3 months; about one-quarter (27%) are using no method of birth control 3 months after stopping OCs

---

References

1. Henshaw SK. Unintended pregnancy in the United States. *Fam Plann Perspect* 1998;30:24-29,46.

2. Trussell J, Vaughan B. Contraceptive failure, method-related discontinuation, and resumption of use: results from the 1995 National Survey of Family Growth. *Fam Plann Perspect* 1999;31:64-72,93.

3. Rosenberg MJ, Waugh MS, Meehan TE. Use and misuse of oral contraceptives: risk indicators for poor pill taking and discontinuation. *Contraception* 1995;51:283-288.

4. Rosenberg MJ, Waugh MS. Oral contraceptive discontinuation: a prospective evaluation of frequency and reasons. *Am J Obstet Gynecol* 1998;179:577-582.

4.1: Special Patient Populations

i. Adolescents

In the United States, many women begin sexual activity during their adolescent years and will need counseling about contraception and prevention of sexually transmitted diseases. Teenagers often delay seeking medical contraception until after they have initiated intercourse; many teens fear contraception or worry that their parents may discover they are sexually active.

Oral contraceptives can be used successfully by teens. As with adults, teens need accurate information about the benefits and risks of the pill, correct use, and side effects. Adolescents may need special counseling, however, about issues such as weight gain, acne, and the use of condoms for STD prevention. Counseling considerations also include uncovering fears and misinformation about OCs communicated by friends and parents, as well as the media. Interactive communication can help the clinician learn more about the teenager's individual situation and help to enhance successful use.

Teen Sexual Activity

Data from the National Survey of Family Growth (NSFG) indicate that the proportion of adolescent women who ever had sexual intercourse increased during the 1980s, but stabilized from 1988 through 1995.[1] The 1982, 1988, and 1995 surveys found that about 40% of all 15- to 19-year-olds had had sexual intercourse during the past 3 months. Among never-married adolescents 15 to 19 years of age, about 45% had had sexual intercourse at least once. Although the percentage having had sexual intercourse declined between 1988 and 1995, the small drop was not statistically significant.

The 1997 Youth Risk Behavior Survey, developed and administered by the Centers for Disease Control and Prevention, also reports that many teens engage in behaviors that place them at high risk for pregnancy and STDs.[2] Among 9th to 12th grade students, about half (48%) have had sexual intercourse. Of those who were sexually active, 43% reported not using a condom at last intercourse (Figure 40).

Figure 40

Percentage of High School Students Participating in Selected Health Risk Behaviors—Youth Risk Behavior Survey, 1997

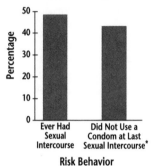

Risk Behavior

*Among currently sexually active students

Source: Centers for Disease Control and Prevention, 1998 (see reference 2).

Initiation of Contraceptive Use

The majority of adolescents delay seeking medical contraceptive services until after they initiate sexual intercourse. Only about 40% of adolescents seek medical contraceptive services within the first year of becoming sexually active.[3]

Delay may occur for several reasons. For example, adolescents may not perceive themselves at risk for an unintended pregnancy. Other reasons for delay include the fear of a pelvic exam or the fear that parents will discover that the adolescent is sexually active.

One study found that the perception of birth control as dangerous contributes to delay.[4] The study of junior and senior high school students found participants' perceptions regarding birth control were more important than cost or ignorance of a source of contraception. Among sexually active teens, the most important reasons given at baseline for not accessing services were fear that contraception is dangerous, cited by 40%; fear of parental discovery, cited by 31%; and awaiting "closer" partner relationships, cited by 31%. A fourth reason teens delayed accessing services was fear of the physical examination. As many as 23% of the young women gave this reason for not obtaining contraception. These reasons were so compelling that even after exposure to an intensive program offering contraceptive counseling services, the sexually active young women who still had not sought contraceptive assistance continued to give these reasons as primary explanations for their delay.

This study lends support to the belief that unwarranted fear of contraception can influence the choice of whether or not to practice birth control. Teenagers are exposed to sexual issues through the media. Although adept at portraying a glamorized representation of sex, the media are reluctant to run ads about birth control, STDs, and AIDS prevention. This makes it particularly important to counsel teenagers (and all women) about the comparative risks of each method, emphasizing the health benefits that may be conferred by the method, and the importance of protecting oneself against unwanted pregnancy and STDs.

Contraceptive Choice at First Intercourse

In 1982, less than 50% of women aged 15 to 19 years used a contraceptive method at first intercourse.[5] This rose to 65% in 1988 and to 77% in 1995.[6,7] According to the NSFG, teens engaging in sexual intercourse for the first time who use a contraceptive method typically choose the condom.[6,7] In fact, the use of a condom doubled from 1982 to 1988, increasing from 23% to 47%. Data from the 1995 NSFG indicate that use of condoms at first intercourse is most likely among teens under 16 years of age (34%).

According to the NSFG, the use of OCs at sexual initiation has declined from about 22% among women who first had sex between 1980 and 1984 to 16% among those initiating intercourse between 1990 and 1995 (Figure 41).[7] The trend is even more pronounced when examining the experience of those who engaged in first intercourse between 1990 and 1995.

Figure 41

Birth Control Method Used at First Intercourse by Year of Sexual Initiation

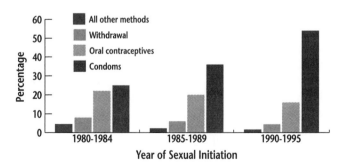

Source: Abma JC, et al, 1997 (see reference 7).

The Hidden Agenda

Teens may visit the clinician with contraception in mind, but not feel comfortable communicating their health needs. Clinicians need to be aware of the possible hidden agenda—many young women will complain of menstrual cramps when they really want birth control pills because they heard that oral contraceptives are commonly prescribed for this indication.

Compliance among Teens

Teenagers present a special challenge because they often do not understand how important it is to take OCs exactly as prescribed. Teens may have more trouble taking OCs correctly than older women, and many teenage pill users quit after a relatively brief period of time.

The 1995 NSFG found that among teens 15 to 17 years of age, 28% reported missing two or more pills in the previous 3 months of OC use. Among older teens, 13% reported missing two or more pills in the 3 months prior.[7] These data indicate that counseling about proper OC use may be particularly important among younger teens. Recent onset of OC use and a previous unintended pregnancy were also associated with higher rates of inconsistent OC use.[8]

Clinicians must dispel myths, such as the belief that the pill causes weight gain or leads to lasting infertility or birth defects. For example, one myth among many pill takers is that protection against pregnancy persists for some months after stopping the pill.

Teens may particularly benefit from verbal instruction about OC use because written instructions may be discarded because of fear of parental discovery. On the other hand, when parental knowledge is not a concern, involving the teen's parents may enhance compliance.

Clinicians should encourage teens to ask questions before they leave the office or clinic. Teens should be urged to call immediately if any questions arise—rather than consulting friends. The name and phone number of the health care provider to call should be given to the patient and she should meet the staff member in person, if possible. In addition, practitioners may wish to schedule more frequent visits with teenage patients than with adults.

Other compliance problems concern logistical factors for teens who may be limited by their health plans or may only have enough money to get 1 month's supply at a time. Sunday-start pills may also be a problem for those who run out over the weekend and may not be able to contact their prescribers to obtain a refill.

One other reason given for discontinuation is inconvenience. Although the pill is a fairly convenient method of contraception, adolescents (as well as adults) may have chaotic schedules. This is particularly true if a teenager's parents are divorced and she is spending weekends at a different home or, in the case of an older teen, if she is away at school.

Anticipatory Counseling about Side Effects

Misperceptions and concerns about possible side effects may deter OC use and contribute to noncompliance and OC discontinuation. Teens who experience breakthrough bleeding or amenorrhea are more concerned than those who do not. Breakthrough bleeding may lead to increased anxiety, disruption of sexual relations, and having to use more tampons or pads, which can be an issue in high school, where teens may have 5 minutes to change classes and run to the bathroom.

Teens have many concerns about OCs, which can vary among populations (Figure 42).[9] Suburban teens are overwhelmingly concerned about weight gain, an issue which needs to be addressed the first time oral contraceptives are discussed. Inner-city teens are concerned about weight gain, too, but may also have fears about blood clots, birth defects, and infertility. Practitioners should dispel misconceptions regarding the pill to help improve compliance.

Also, appointments for adolescents who are at high risk for teen pregnancy should be flexible. Teens who have school failure or who are the siblings of parenting teens are at greater risk of noncompliance. If the patient has a teenage sister who is either pregnant and carrying to term or a parenting teen, that teenager is at high risk of an unplanned pregnancy. Young people who have sexually transmitted diseases, who have multiple (or serial) partners, or who are involved in substance abuse also need to be seen more frequently.

Figure 42

Concerns Expressed about Oral Contraceptives by Teens in an Adolescent Clinic and in Private Practice

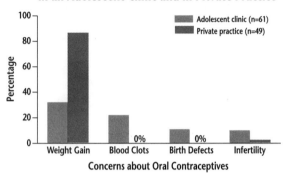

Source: Emans SJ, et al, 1987 (see reference 9).

Parents' Perceptions

Parents of teens may also have negative attitudes about oral contraception. In one Canadian study, mothers were the source of contraceptive information for 15% of teens.[10] The mothers of many teenagers today are familiar with the pills that were available in the '60s and '70s—pills that were high dose and caused more nuisance side effects, such as nausea. During the '70s, substantial negative media coverage surrounded the pill. So, parents of today's teens may be giving their daughters obsolete information.

Strategies for STD Protection

Condom use needs to be discussed with adolescents, particularly young women who are choosing to use the pill or other hormonal methods. Clinicians can open the discussion by asking, "Does your boyfriend use condoms? If not, how could you get him to use them? Will he continue to use condoms after you go on the pill?" Clinicians should counsel teens about the pros and cons of sharing the initiation of OC use with their partners if it might impact the decision to use condoms.

Condom counseling is particularly important with younger patients. Adolescents who use hormonal methods of contraception may be less likely to use condoms than other sexually active teens.[11]

However, educational interventions aimed at promoting condom use can substantially increase the proportion of teens who simultaneously use OCs and condoms. In one randomized controlled trial, 383 African-American adolescents attended a series of counseling sessions that included information about STDs, HIV, and contraception. The number of OC users who also used condoms increased approximately 20%.[12]

Delay of Pelvic Exam

In 1993, the FDA changed package insert labeling such that a pelvic examination is no longer required before prescribing oral contraceptives. Following its Fertility and Maternal Health Drugs advisory committee recommendation, the FDA decided to remove the pelvic exam requirement because it could limit OC access for many women. The new labeling reads, "Physical examination may be deferred until after initiation of oral contraceptives if requested by the woman and judged appropriate by the clinician." Three situations exist for which women seeking OCs might want to defer the pelvic exam. One, teenagers may avoid going to the clinic or physician's office due to fear of the examination. Two, women seeking contraception may have an appointment during their menstrual period and may have to reschedule. Three, some women who wish to use OCs may have a long delay in scheduling an appointment that would include time for the complete physical examination. ACOG and the American Society for Reproductive Medicine support the FDA's recommendation.

While the pelvic exam can be deferred, it should be performed as part of comprehensive preventive services for teens. *The Guidelines for Adolescent Preventive Services* and the *Bright Futures Guidelines* both recommend a pelvic examination for sexually active teens.[13,14]

Contraceptive Counseling

The Initial Interview

To enhance compliance with contraception, clinicians ideally should learn about the teenager's general health, her psychosocial and family history, and her goals for the future.[15] Start the interview slowly and gain the patient's trust. Begin with less sensitive areas—what is going on at school or what she enjoys doing in her leisure time. This will help the clinician develop a relationship with the teen and, hopefully, enhance her trust and confidence. Then, the clinician can move on to the patient's reproductive health history and sexual behavior. Ask a patient what she knows about a particular topic—STDs, for example—rather than give a prepared talk.

Confidentiality

The issue of confidentiality is very important for adolescent patients.[16,17] One study reported that 58% of adolescents had health concerns they did not want shared with their parents.[16] A quarter of the adolescents surveyed reported that they would not seek health services in some situations if their parents might be informed (Figure 43). Another survey of high school students in Massachusetts also found that adolescents who knew that their doctors provided confidential care were about three times more likely to discuss sexuality-related issues than teens who did not believe their care was confidential.[18]

Parental Involvement

Parental knowledge and support may enhance compliance with contraception, especially for the young teen. The American

Figure 43

Perceptions of Adolescents Regarding Confidentiality Issues

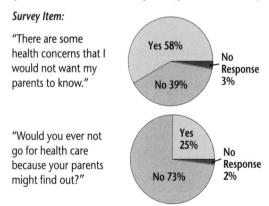

Survey Item:

"There are some health concerns that I would not want my parents to know."

Yes 58%
No Response 3%
No 39%

"Would you ever not go for health care because your parents might find out?"

Yes 25%
No Response 2%
No 73%

Source: Cheng TL, et al, 1993 (see reference 16).

Academy of Pediatrics recommends involving parents, when possible. Teens should be encouraged to share their decision to use hormonal contraception with their parents, but confidentiality is important for those who do not feel comfortable doing so. Many teens are more comfortable sharing about their use of OCs for medical reasons, such as acne, dysmenorrhea, or irregular menses.

Take Home Messages

- Among never-married adolescents 15 to 19 years old, about half have had sexual intercourse at least once

- Many teens fear contraception is dangerous

- Adolescents may have a "hidden agenda"—seeking medical services for menstrual cramps or other reasons when they are hoping to receive a prescription for OCs

- The 1997 Youth Risk Behavior Survey indicates that 43% of teenagers reported not using a condom at last intercourse

- Teenagers using OCs need counseling about condom use for STD prevention

---

References

1. Singh S, Darroch JE. Trends in sexual activity among adolescent American women: 1982-1995. *Fam Plann Perspect* 1999;31:212-219.

2. Centers for Disease Control and Prevention. Youth Risk Behavior Surveillance—United States, 1997. *MMWR* 1998;47(SS-3):1-89.

3. The Alan Guttmacher Institute. *Sex and America's Teenagers.* New York, NY: The Alan Guttmacher Institute; 1994.

4. Zabin LS, Stark HA, Emerson MR. Reasons for delay in contraceptive clinic utilization. *J Adolesc Health* 1991;12:225-232.

5. Mosher WD, Bachrach CA. First premarital contraceptive use: United States, 1960-1982. *Stud Fam Plann* 1987;18:83-95.

6. Forrest JD, Singh S. The sexual and reproductive behavior of American women, 1982-1988. *Fam Plann Perspect* 1990;22:206-214.

7. Abma JC, Chandra A, Mosher WD, et al. Fertility, family planning, and women's health: new data from the 1995 National Survey of Family Growth. National Center for Health Statistics. *Vital Health Stat* 1997;23(19).

8. Peterson LS, Oakley D, Potter LS, et al. Women's efforts to prevent pregnancy: consistency of oral contraceptive use. *Fam Plann Perspect* 1998; 30:19-23.

9. Emans SJ, Grace E, Woods ER, et al. Adolescents' compliance with the use of oral contraceptives. *JAMA* 1987;257:3377-3381.

10. Herold ES, Goodwin MS. Perceived side effects of oral contraceptives among adolescent girls. *Can Med Assoc J* 1980;123:1022-1026.

11. Roye CF. Condom use by Hispanic and African-American adolescent girls who use hormonal contraception. *J Adolesc Health* 1998;23:205-211.

12. Stanton BF, Li X, Galbraith J, et al. Sexually transmitted diseases, human immunodeficiency virus, and pregnancy prevention. *Arch Pediatr Adolesc Med* 1996;150:17-24.

13. American Medical Association. *Guidelines for Adolescent Preventive Services. Recommendations Monograph.* Chicago, IL: American Medical Association; 1996.

14. Green M, ed. *Bright Futures—Guidelines for Health Supervision of Infants, Children, and Adolescents.* Arlington, VA: National Center for Education in Maternal and Child Health; 1994.

15. Neinstein LS. The office visit and interview techniques. In: *Adolescent Health Care: A Practical Guide.* Baltimore, MD: Williams & Wilkins; 1991.

16. Cheng TL, Savageau JA, Sattler AL, et al. Confidentiality in health care: a survey of knowledge, perceptions, and attitudes among high school students. *JAMA* 1993;269:1404-1407.

17. Ford CA, Millstein SG, Halpern-Felsher BL, et al. Influence of physician confidentiality assurances on adolescent willingness to disclose information and seek future health care: randomized controlled trial. *JAMA* 1997;278: 1029-1034.

18. Thrall JS, McCloskey L, Rothstein E, et al. Perception of confidentiality and adolescents' use of health care services and information. Society for Adolescent Medicine Annual Meeting; March 7, 1997, San Francisco, CA. Poster presentation.

ii. Women over Age 35 Years

In early 1990, the FDA accepted the recommendation of its Fertility and Maternal Health Drugs Advisory Committee to revise the labeling for oral contraceptives. In a letter to manufacturers, the FDA requested that the language of the patient information be modified.[1] Specifically, reference to increased cardiovascular mortality risks among healthy, non-smoking women aged 40 years and older was deleted. Changing demographics have created an upsurge in the number of women in their later reproductive years. These women and their clinicians need to know that OCs can be a safe and effective option.

The benefits of OCs for healthy, nonsmoking women over age 35 years outweigh the risks. Furthermore, the pill provides many noncontraceptive benefits that must be weighed against possible risks. Although the FDA has never identified age as a mandatory contraindication to OC use, earlier labeling often determined *de facto* age limits—limits adhered to by physicians unwilling to prescribe outside of labeling.

Since 1985, ACOG has taken the position that low-dose OCs are safe and appropriate contraception for healthy, nonsmoking women over age 35 years.[2] Low-dose OCs, the most widely used preparations today, are effective and cause few side effects.[3]

Origins of Age Limitations

The original data from the Royal College of General Practitioners' Oral Contraception Study found an increased risk of death from vascular disease with increasing duration of OC use.[4] Other studies published in 1975 found that OC users were at increased risk of fatal and nonfatal myocardial infarction. The risk was elevated among women aged 30 to 39 years and increased more among women aged 40 to 44 years.[5,6]

These early studies were eventually reanalyzed and the risk of myocardial infarction initially attributed to OCs was determined to be largely the result of a critical confounding factor—smoking. Unfortunately, the delayed recognition of the smoking factor led to a distorted perception of the safety of OCs, particularly among women in their later reproductive years.

Current OC Use

The 1995 NSFG documents low utilization of the pill among women 35 years and older using contraception.[7] Among women aged 20 to 24 years, about 54% use the pill. OC use declines until, at age 35 years, the percentage of women who use OCs is less than 10%. For women aged 40 to 44 years, the percentage using the pill is 6%. Although these data clearly indicate that OC use is uncommon among older women, OC use has increased substantially among women over age 35 years since 1982, doubling among women 35 to 39 years of age and increasing sixfold among women 40 to 44 years of age.

Unintended Pregnancy

Safe, effective contraception is important for women in their later reproductive years as the risk of genetic abnormalities increases and the high abortion ratio indicates many conceptions are unwanted. The 1995 NSFG found that 51% of pregnancies to women 40 years of age or older were unintended; about 60% of these unplanned pregnancies ended in induced abortion.[8] Besides preventing unintended pregnancies, OCs can prove helpful in maintaining regular bleeding cycles and a consistent hormonal pattern up to menopause.

Screening

Current recommendations concerning screening women age 40 years and older when prescribing OCs vary among practitioners and health organizations. Recommendations differ, depending upon family history of cardiovascular disease, diabetes, age, and cigarette smoking. Healthy, nonsmoking women aged 40 years and older do not need additional screening prior to use of low-dose OCs.

Switching to Hormone Replacement Therapy

If women wish to switch to hormone replacement therapy, it is advisable not to discontinue oral contraceptives in order to attempt to diagnose menopause. If the woman is still premenopausal, stopping OCs unnecessarily may put her at risk of an unintended pregnancy. Additionally, women who truly are menopausal will potentially endure unnecessary vasomotor symptoms.

A study of 24 menopausal women given low-dose OCs demonstrated that laboratory testing can be performed on day 7 of the placebo week to identify menopause.[9] Simply measuring follicle-stimulating hormone (FSH) levels is insufficient, as only 38% of menopausal women have a serum FSH $\geq$30 mIU/mL 7 days after discontinuing low-dose OCs. The study demonstrated that an FSH:LH [luteinizing hormone] ratio >1 is present in 100% of women, and serum estradiol levels are <25 pg/mL in 90% of women, by this time. Thus, these tests can suggest the diagnosis of menopause without having the patient discontinue oral contraceptives.[9]

Take Home Messages

- *Low-dose OCs can provide safe, effective contraception for healthy, nonsmoking women over age 35 years up to menopause*

Continued on next page

Take Home Messages (continued)

- *Benefits of OCs for this age group include the maintenance of a consistent hormonal pattern during the perimenopause and potential for preservation of bone mineral density*
- *In women over 35 years of age, use of OCs is uncommon, but is increasing*

References

1. F-D-C Reports. *The Pink Sheet.* February 5, 1990;T&G-8.

2. American College of Obstetricians and Gynecologists. Contraception for women in their later reproductive years. *ACOG Committee Opinion* 1985;41.

3. Mishell DR Jr. Contraception. *N Engl J Med* 1989;320:777-787.

4. Beral V. Mortality among oral contraceptive users: Royal College of General Practitioners' Oral Contraception Study. *Lancet* 1977;2:727.

5. Mann JI, Vessey MP, Thorogood M, et al. Myocardial infarction in young women with special reference to oral contraceptive practice. *BMJ* 1975;2: 241-244.

6. Mann JI, Inman WHW. Oral contraceptives and death from myocardial infarction. *BMJ* 1975;2:245.

7. Piccinino LJ, Mosher WD. Trends in contraceptive use in the United States: 1982-1995. *Fam Plann Perspect* 1998;30:4-10,46.

8. Henshaw SK. Unintended pregnancy in the United States. *Fam Plann Perspect* 1998;30:24-29,46.

9. Creinin MD. Laboratory criteria for menopause in women using oral contraceptives. *Fertil Steril* 1996;66:101-104.

iii. Breastfeeding Women

Patients who plan to breastfeed need to be counseled regarding choice of contraceptive method, preferably before giving birth. Another appropriate time for additional contraceptive counseling is just prior to hospital discharge. Combination or progestin-only oral contraceptives can be appropriate choices. No evidence exists that low-dose combined OCs affect breast milk production or carbohydrate content, nor that they impair infant growth, development, or intelligence.

Progestin-Only OCs

Progestin-only oral contraceptives ("mini-pills") can be used in combination with breastfeeding. A small amount of hormone passes into the breast milk, but has no known adverse effects on the infant. In addition, certain progestins provide a modest boost to milk production; at least one study has shown that women using progestin-only pills (POPs) breastfed longer and added supplementary feeding at a later date.[1] The timing of POP initiation in breastfeeding women continues to be debated. In general, women who are exclusively breastfeeding may begin POPs 6 weeks after giving birth. (For further discussion, see the section on progestin-only OCs.)

Combination OCs

Combination OCs containing both estrogen and progestin are another option. Both estrogen and progestin may pass from the mother to the infant through breast milk. Both ACOG and the American Academy of Pediatrics approve the use of combination oral contraceptives in women electing to breastfeed once lactation is well established.[2,3]

Studies of *high-dose* OCs have shown that the milk supply is decreased in women who use combination OCs. Although milk output and composition may have been affected by use of high-dose OCs, these effects did not hurt infant growth or health.[4,5] The longest follow-up study has been of Swedish children whose mothers used combination OCs while nursing. No adverse effects have been found on the physical, intellectual, or psychological development of these children.[6]

The World Health Organization suggests that combination OCs should not be the first-choice method for lactating women. The conservative recommendations with regard to breastfeeding women and combined OCs are controversial, however, because of the lack of evidence of any adverse effect of low-dose OCs.

Although combination OCs are appropriate for women once lactation has been established, some clinicians prefer the use of a nonhormonal method or the mini-pill for women who are breastfeeding. If combination OCs are chosen, they can be started about 6 weeks postpartum. Controversy exists over the risk for thromboembolic events when using combination OCs immediately after childbirth.[7] Low-dose pills may have less of an effect on the risk for thromboembolism than higher-dose formulations.

Take Home Messages

- *Progestin-only and combined OCs are both options for breast-feeding women*

- *The American Academy of Pediatrics has approved the use of combination OCs in breastfeeding women once lactation is well established*

- *No evidence exists that low-dose combined OCs affect breast milk production, carbohydrate content, infant growth, psychological development, or intelligence*

- *Among nursing women, combination OCs can be started about 6 weeks postpartum*

- *In general, women who are exclusively breastfeeding may begin progestin-only OCs 6 weeks after giving birth*

References

1. McCann MF, Moggia AV, Higgins JE, et al. The effects of a progestin-only oral contraceptive (levonorgestrel 0.03 mg) on breast-feeding. *Contraception* 1989;40:635-648.

2. American College of Obstetricians and Gynecologists. Hormonal contraception. *ACOG Technical Bulletin* 1994;198.

3. American Academy of Pediatrics. The transfer of drugs and other chemicals into human milk (RE9403). *Pediatrics* 1994;93:137-150.

4. WHO Special Programme of Research, Development, and Research Training in Human Reproduction, Task Force on Oral Contraceptives. Effects of hormonal contraceptives on milk volume and infant growth. *Contraception* 1984;30:505-522.

5. WHO Special Programme of Research, Development, and Research Training in Human Reproduction, Task Force on Oral Contraceptives. Effects of hormonal contraceptives on breast milk composition and infant growth. *Stud Fam Plann* 1988;19:361-369.

6. Nilsson S, Mellbin T, Hofvander Y, et al. Long-term follow-up of children breast-fed by mothers using oral contraceptives. *Contraception* 1986;34: 443-457.

7. WHO Task Force on Oral Contraceptives. Contraceptives during the postpartum period and during lactation: the effects on women's health. *Int J Gynecol Obstet* 1987;25S:13-27.

iv. Mentally Handicapped

Women with limited mental capacity have a broad range of sexual and reproductive needs.[1,2] Among these are sex education, socialization skills, knowledge of appropriate "private" versus "public" behaviors, and strategies to avoid sexual abuse. Counseling concerning contraception, sterilization, and STDs also may be warranted. While these socialization and sexuality concerns are typical among women of normal intelligence, various intellectual, social, and educational deficits complicate these issues for those who are mentally handicapped.[2,3]

All women with mental handicaps face a number of challenges in dealing with social and sexual development, often requiring special attention to help them cope with physical changes and developing sexuality. Women with mental handicaps can be especially vulnerable to sexual exploitation, particularly those who are affectionate or unknowingly exhibit seductive behavior.[4] Often, these young women are socialized to be dependent and respectful of authority, which may also increase their vulnerability.

Chamberlain et al reported that the incidence of sexual abuse is highest among mildly retarded adolescents.[5] The study of 87 women found that one-third of mildly retarded and one-fourth of moderately retarded adolescents had been victims of rape or incest. In most cases, the assailant was a family member or someone whom the victim knew well.

Contraception

Women with mental handicaps have unique needs for contraception.[1,3,4] One obstacle to contraception is the reluctance of parents, other caregivers, or health care providers to acknowledge the sexuality and sexual needs of persons with mental handicaps.[4] Despite limitations of cognitive development, mentally handicapped adolescents reach sexual maturation at about the same time as other adolescents and often display curiosity about sex and sexual feelings.

A study of adolescent women with mental disabilities found that about 50% had had sexual intercourse.[5] Among the moderately retarded adolescents, 32% were sexually active. Importantly, of the 14 young women who were sexually active, 43% became pregnant.

The high rate of unintended pregnancy suggests a need for adequate and appropriate sex education and information about contraception.

Clinicians should assess several factors before recommending a contraceptive method. The woman's understanding and reasons for participating in sexual intercourse need to be evaluated. Does she understand what she is doing? Is she a willing participant? Other considerations include the predicted frequency of intercourse, the patient's ability to use the method, and the anticipated circumstances under which intercourse is likely to occur.[3]

In general, OCs are a good method, provided that compliance is not a concern and that the woman has no contraindicating medical problems. OCs have the benefits of decreasing menstrual flow, reducing dysmenorrhea, and establishing predictable menstrual cycles. Clinicians prescribing OCs should encourage the caretaker to make sure the pill is taken every day.[4]

Long-acting methods requiring little compliance, such as implants, DMPA, and the IUD, have advantages in this population. The potential for amenorrhea makes DMPA a particularly appealing choice. Especially for women with other physical problems, the benefits of effective contraception must always be weighed against the risks of pregnancy to both the woman and fetus.[6]

Take Home Messages

- *Adolescent and adult women with limited mental capacity may need contraception and counseling about STDs*

- *OCs can be a good choice, especially if the caregiver can make sure the medication is taken every day*

- *Advantages of OCs for women with mental disabilities include reduced menstrual flow, relief of dysmenorrhea, and predictable menstrual cycles*

References

1. Haefner HK, Elkins TE. Contraceptive management for female adolescents with mental retardation and handicapping disabilities. *Curr Opin Obstet Gynecol* 1991;3:820-824.

2. Elkins TE, Kope S, Ghaziuddin M, et al. Integration of a sexuality counseling service into a reproductive health program for persons with mental retardation. *J Pediatr Adolesc Gynecol* 1997;10:24-27.

3. Hein K, Coupey SM, Cohen MI. Special considerations in pregnancy prevention for the mentally subnormal adolescent female. *J Adolesc Health Care* 1980;1:46-49.

4. Kreutner AK. Sexuality, fertility, and the problems of menstruation in mentally retarded adolescents. *Pediatr Clin North Am* 1981;28:475-480.

5. Chamberlain A, Rauh J, Passer A, et al. Issues in fertility control for mentally retarded female adolescents: I. Sexual activity, sexual abuse, and contraception. *Pediatrics* 1984;73:445-450.

6. Mattson RH, Cramer JA, Darney PD, et al. Use of oral contraceptives by women with epilepsy. *JAMA* 1986;256:238-240.

v. Women with Medical Disorders

Women in their reproductive years with medical disorders have special needs with regard to contraception. Many medical conditions preclude pregnancy because they can cause serious complications in pregnancy or because pregnancy can aggravate existing medical problems. Therefore, the need to plan pregnancies and prevent unwanted pregnancies is even greater for these women than for healthy women.

Health care providers are often unsure of the best approach to contraception for women with medical disorders. Because most studies of contraceptives are limited to healthy women, the lack of available data regarding the effects of a chosen contraceptive method upon a particular disease make it difficult to know the risks of exacerbating an illness. As a result, clinicians may refuse to offer a contraceptive method because they lack information about the consequences of pregnancy and the effects of a method on the disease.

However, by acting out of the fear of the *error of commission*, health care providers may commit the *error of omission*. The former involves prescribing a method that results in complications for the patient and the possibility of legal action. The latter involves withholding an effective contraceptive method and increasing the likelihood of a high-risk pregnancy.

Health providers need to conduct a risk-benefit analysis when recommending contraception to women with health problems. Jones and Wild developed a formula to assist clinicians and patients in evaluating a contraceptive method (Figure 44).[1] The formula depends upon assessing information from four areas: the risk of exacerbation of the disease, the risk of pregnancy, patient factors, and the effectiveness of the method.

Figure 44

Risk Analysis Formula

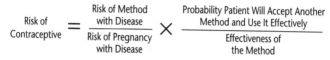

Source: Jones KP, Wild R. Contraception for patients with psychiatric or medical disorders. Am J Obstet Gynecol 1994;170:1575-1580. Reproduced with permission of Mosby, Inc.

Clinicians should assess patient factors that influence the decision to use a method and consider the effectiveness of the method. Patient factors include risk-taking behavior and plans for future pregnancy. The patient's ability and willingness to use a method consistently and effectively must be taken into consideration. For example, if the patient does not think she will use a diaphragm consistently, then this method may not be an appropriate choice, even if it is considered safe. Effectiveness of the method also will influence contraceptive choice. The greater the risk of a pregnancy, the more desirable it is to use a highly effective method.

The formula gives practitioners a way to evaluate the appropriateness of a method. A method of contraception is appropriate when the risks of pregnancy are greater than the possible risks of the contraceptive method and the patient is unlikely to use another method effectively. Special considerations, such as manual dexterity, the presence of a bleeding disorder, or possible interaction with other medications, must also be taken into account.

Many clinicians fear using hormonal methods in women with medical problems. However, if hormones can exacerbate a woman's disease, then pregnancy may exacerbate the illness to an even greater degree. Women should not automatically be excluded from using OCs because they have medical problems. With a proper evaluation of the risks and benefits and informed decision-making, the pill can be an appropriate option for many women with medical disorders.

Take Home Messages

- *Women with medical disorders often have special needs concerning contraception*
- *If hormones are suspected to exacerbate an illness, then pregnancy may exacerbate the condition to an even greater degree*
- *Clinicians need to consider the patient's willingness to use the method, the effectiveness of the method, and the risks of pregnancy*

Reference
1. Jones KP, Wild RA. Contraception for patients with psychiatric or medical disorders. *Am J Obstet Gynecol* 1994;170:1575-1580.

4.2: Sexually Transmitted Disease

Oral contraceptives help protect against pelvic inflammatory disease (PID) requiring hospitalization, a common complication of STD infection; OC users are about half as likely to develop the condition as nonusers. On the other hand, OC users are at greater risk for detection of chlamydial cervical infection. Condoms remain the most important means of preventing STDs and HIV in women at risk.

STDs and HIV are a major public health challenge in the United States (Figure 45). Despite reductions in the rates of gonorrhea and syphilis in recent years, the US has the highest rates of STD infection in the industrialized world—as much as 50 to 100 times higher than other industrialized nations.[1] Furthermore, STD infection is disproportionately high among teenagers and minorities. Of the 12 million new cases of STDs each year in the US, 3 million occur among individuals aged 13 to 19 years.[1]

Women bear a disproportionate share of the impact of STDs. Serious complications include PID, infertility, ectopic pregnancy, cancer of the reproductive tract, adverse pregnancy outcome,

Figure 45

Estimated Number of New STD Cases or Infections Annually in the US

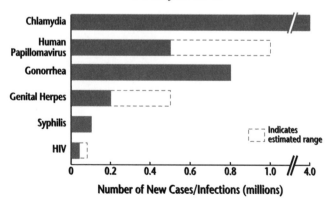

Number of New Cases/Infections (millions)

Source: Centers for Disease Control and Prevention, 1996 (see reference 1).

infant pneumonia, and infant death. STDs also play an integral role in the transmission of HIV; genital ulcers can increase the likelihood that HIV exposure will result in infection.

Protection Against PID

Upper genital tract infection is a frequent complication of two of the most common STDs, chlamydia and gonorrhea. If not properly treated, 20% to 40% of women with chlamydia and 10% to 40% of women with gonorrhea will develop PID. Among women who develop PID, about 20% will suffer involuntary infertility as a result of scarring. Nearly one-fifth will endure chronic pelvic pain. Another 9% will experience ectopic pregnancy, the leading cause of first trimester maternal mortality in the US.[2]

OCs are associated with a reduced risk of hospitalization for PID.[3-5] (For further discussion, see the section on health benefits.)

Whether OC protection against PID varies by infecting pathogen is unclear. In a case-control study that evaluated relative risk of PID among OC users according to infecting organism (*Chlamydia trachomatis* or *Neisseria gonorrhoeae*), researchers reported significant protection only among women infected with chlamydia (RR=0.2; 95% CI, 0.1-0.6). OC users with gonorrhea appeared no more or less likely to develop PID than nonusers (Figure 46).[5]

Questions remain as to whether OC use makes women more susceptible to specific infections that can cause PID. Some research has suggested that OC use is associated with a higher risk of chlamydial cervicitis.[6,7] However, these findings may reflect enhanced detection of the pathogen

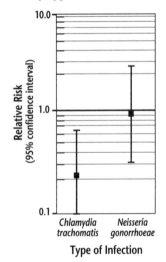

Figure 46

Relative Risk of PID among OC Users vs Nonusers by Type of Infection

Source: Wolner-Hanssen P, et al, 1990 (see reference 5).

in OC users. Researchers have theorized that the higher prevalence of chlamydia reported in OC users may be the result of more efficient collection of cervical specimens from the increased area of the cervical ectropion (resulting from OC use) accessible to collection.[8]

Relationship to HIV

A recent review examined more than 30 studies to determine whether hormonal contraception affects HIV risk.[9] More than 20 of the studies were cross-sectional or retrospective analyses subject to numerous biases. The relative risks varied widely and few achieved statistical significance (Figure 47).[10-17] A tendency also existed for higher odds ratios to be reported in higher-risk women (prostitutes) and lower odds ratios in women attending family planning, antenatal, or other health services.[9]

The evidence concerning combined OCs and HIV is weak. A wide range of associations between protective and harmful have been reported in a variety of populations. These inconsistent results do not allow firm conclusions. One unanswered question is whether hormonal contraception affects the infectiousness of HIV-positive users. Although several studies in Africa have examined hormonal contraceptive use and the degree of HIV shedding in the genital tract, the results are conflicting. Many of the confidence intervals are wide and the studies have relatively small samples.[9]

Long-Acting Progestins

Long-acting progestin methods have been associated with an increased risk of simian immunodeficiency virus infection in monkeys.[18] Researchers hypothesize that progesterone decreases the efficacy of the vaginal barrier by thinning the vaginal epithelium. However, few data exist from human studies; those that do exist are inconclusive.[11,13,17,19]

A National Institutes of Health (NIH) consensus panel reviewed the progestin data in June 1996 and concluded that better human studies were needed. The panel did not recommend any change in prescribing, but emphasized use of condoms for STD/HIV prevention in women at risk.

Two large, ongoing studies should help provide more definitive answers in the near future. These studies are gathering data on

Figure 47

Risk of HIV Transmission to Women Using Hormonal Contraceptives: Recent Prospective Studies

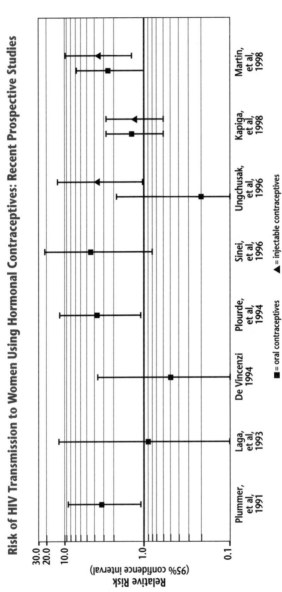

Sources: Adapted from references 10-17.

hormonal contraception and HIV—one on injectable progestins that the Centers for Disease Control and Prevention is conducting in South Africa and another on combined oral and injectable contraceptives that the NIH and Family Health International are conducting in Thailand, Uganda, and Zimbabwe. These data should be available in 2002.

Take Home Messages

- *OCs decrease the risk of PID requiring hospitalization*
- *OC users may be at greater risk for chlamydial cervicitis; however, these findings may reflect enhanced detection of the pathogen or more efficient collection of cervical specimens*
- *Evidence concerning combined OCs and HIV is weak; no firm conclusions can be drawn*
- *Whether hormonal contraception affects the infectiousness of HIV-positive users is unknown*
- *Clinicians should emphasize the use of condoms for STD prevention in women at risk*

References

1. Centers for Disease Control and Prevention. Division of STD Prevention. *The Challenge of STD Prevention in the United States.* Atlanta: Centers for Disease Control and Prevention, November 1996.

2. Centers for Disease Control and Prevention. Division of STD Prevention. *Sexually Transmitted Disease Surveillance, 1997.* US Department of Health and Human Services, Public Health Service. Atlanta: Centers for Disease Control and Prevention, September 1998.

3. Rubin GL, Ory HW, Layde PM. Oral contraceptives and pelvic inflammatory disease. *Am J Obstet Gynecol* 1982;144:630-635.

4. Wolner-Hanssen P, Svensson L, Mardh PA, et al. Laparoscopic findings and contraceptive use in women with signs and symptoms suggestive of acute salpingitis. *Obstet Gynecol* 1985;66:233-238.

5. Wolner-Hanssen P, Eschenbach DA, Paavonen J, et al. Decreased risk of symptomatic chlamydial pelvic inflammatory disease associated with oral contraceptive use. *JAMA* 1990;263:54-59.

6. Washington AE, Gove S, Schachter J, et al. Oral contraceptives, *Chlamydia trachomatis* infection and pelvic inflammatory disease: a word of caution about protection. *JAMA* 1985;253:2246-2250.

7. Handsfield HJ, Jasman LL, Robert PL, et al. Criteria for selective screening for *Chlamydia trachomatis* infection in women attending family planning clinics. *JAMA* 1986;255:1730-1734.

8. Creatsas G. Sexually transmitted diseases and oral contraceptive use during adolescence. *Ann NY Acad Sci* 1997;816:404-410.

9. Stephenson JM. Systematic review of hormonal contraception and risk of HIV transmission: when to resist meta-analysis. *AIDS* 1998;12:545-553.

10. De Vincenzi I. A longitudinal study of human immunodeficiency virus transmission by heterosexual partners. *N Engl J Med* 1994;331:341-346.

11. Kapiga SH, Lyamuya EF, Lwihula GK, et al. The incidence of HIV infection among women using family planning methods in Dar es Salaam, Tanzania. *AIDS* 1998;12:75-84.

12. Laga M, Manoka A, Kivuvu M, et al. Non-ulcerative sexually transmitted diseases as risk factors for HIV-1 transmission in women: results from a cohort study. *AIDS* 1993;7:95-102.

13. Martin HL Jr, Nyange PM, Richardson BA, et al. Hormonal contraception, sexually transmitted diseases, and risk of heterosexual transmission of human immunodeficiency virus type 1. *J Infect Dis* 1998;178:1053-1059.

14. Plourde PJ, Pepin J, Agoki E, et al. Human immunodeficiency virus type 1 seroconversion in women with genital ulcers. *J Infect Dis* 1994;170:313-317.

15. Plummer FA, Simonsen JN, Cameron DW, et al. Cofactors in male-female sexual transmission of human immunodeficiency virus type 1. *J Infect Dis* 1991;163:233-239.

16. Sinei SKA, Fortney JA, Kigondu CS, et al. Contraceptive use and HIV infection in Kenyan family planning clinic attenders. *Int J STD AIDS* 1996;7:65-70.

17. Ungchusak K, Rehle T, Thammapornpilap P, et al. Determinants of HIV infection among female commercial sex workers in North Eastern Thailand: results from a longitudinal study. *J Acquir Immune Defic Syndr Hum Retrovirol* 1996;12:500-507.

18. Marx PA, Spira AI, Gettie A, et al. Progesterone implants enhance SIV vaginal transmission and early virus load. *Nature Med* 1996;2:1084-1089.

19. Bulterys M, Chao A, Habimana P, et al. Incident HIV-1 infection in a cohort of young women in Butare, Rwanda. *AIDS* 1994;8:1585-1591.

4.3: Hormonal Emergency Contraception

US women and their clinicians have two hormonal emergency contraception options—one contains a combination of levonorgestrel and ethinyl estradiol (PREVEN)* and the other contains levonorgestrel alone (Plan B).* The combination method has been used for many years; however, recent research has shown that levonorgestrel alone is more effective and has fewer side effects.

Plan B Emergency Contraceptive Pills

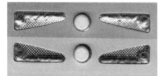

First dose: Take one tablet within 72 hours of unprotected intercourse.

Second dose: Take remaining tablet 12 hours after the first dose.

Plan B (levonorgestrel 0.75 mg)

Source: Adapted from Women's Capitol Corporation.

PREVEN Emergency Contraceptive Kit

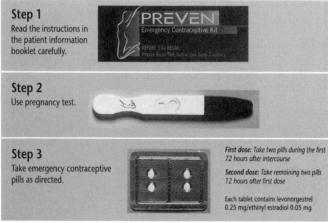

Step 1
Read the instructions in the patient information booklet carefully.

Step 2
Use pregnancy test.

Step 3
Take emergency contraceptive pills as directed.

First dose: *Take two pills during the first 72 hours after intercourse*

Second dose: *Take remaining two pills 12 hours after first dose*

Each tablet contains levonorgestrel 0.25 mg/ethinyl estradiol 0.05 mg

Source: Gynétics Inc.

*Brand names are for identification purposes only and do not imply endorsement.

i. Combination OCs

In late 1998 in the United States, combination emergency contraceptive pills carrying FDA-approved labeling became commercially available.[1] The specially packaged product, the PREVEN™ Emergency Contraceptive Kit, contains four pills of a high-dose combination of ethinyl estradiol and levonorgestrel (the Yuzpe method).

While some OCs were used "off-label" for emergency contraception prior to September 1998, routine use was limited in the US. A survey commissioned by the Henry J. Kaiser Family Foundation of 2,002 US adults found that only 1% said they or their partners had used emergency contraception.[2] A second survey of 307 obstetrician-gynecologists found that although about 70% said they had prescribed emergency contraception within the last year, 77% did so infrequently — five or fewer times.[2]

Easy Packaging

PREVEN packaging makes prescribing and taking emergency contraception more accessible. The kit, which retails for about $20, contains the required medication, a patient education booklet, and a pregnancy test. Each tablet contains 50 µg ethinyl estradiol and 0.25 mg levonorgestrel. Following a negative pregnancy test, two pills should be taken as soon as possible (within 72 hours) after unprotected intercourse or a suspected method failure. A second dose of two pills should be taken 12 hours after the first dose.

Efficacy and Safety Profile

In general, emergency contraceptive pills are less effective than OCs. When used for emergency contraception, the Yuzpe regimen's effectiveness is about 55% to 75%.[3-5]

In the 13 years following the Yuzpe regimen's approval in the United Kingdom, it was used more than 4 million times.[6] Few adverse events were reported: 115 reports of 159 "reactions" (some women reported more than one reaction), 61 of which were pregnancies.[6] Three cerebrovascular events and three venous thromboembolic events were reported.

The relationship of these events to the use of the Yuzpe regimen, if any, is unclear. According to an FDA review prior to endorsing the regimen, "only six serious adverse reactions associated with these products for this use were reported to [the British Medicines Control Agency] from 1984 to 1996. Of these, only one occurred close enough to the time of administration to indicate that the reaction *might* (italics added) be drug related."[7]

The most common side effects are nausea (50%) and vomiting (20%). Less common effects include menstrual irregularities, breast tenderness, headache, abdominal pain, and dizziness.

Reducing Nausea and Vomiting

Nausea and vomiting are unpleasant for women and also increase the chance that women will need an additional dose of medication. Pretreatment with an antiemetic before the initial dose of combination emergency contraception can help alleviate symptoms. A randomized controlled trial found an over-the-counter antiemetic, meclizine, significantly reduced the incidence of nausea and vomiting associated with the Yuzpe method.[8] Investigators randomly assigned 343 women aged 18 to 45 years to pretreatment with meclizine 50 mg, placebo, or no drug 1 hour before the first dose of emergency contraceptive pills. The incidence of nausea was 47% in the group pretreated with meclizine and 64% in the other two groups; however, about twice as many women in the meclizine group reported drowsiness compared to placebo (31% vs 13%, p<0.01).

Contraindications

Both WHO and International Planned Parenthood Federation® find no absolute contraindications to the use of the estrogen/progestin regimen, except known pregnancy. FDA-approved labeling in the US, however, lists clotting problems, ischemic heart disease, stroke, migraine, liver tumors, breast cancer, and past breast biopsies as contraindications. These contraindications are estrogen-related conditions and come from the package labeling for combined oral contraceptives; however, no evidence exists to support these contraindications for short-term therapy with emergency contraception.

Take Home Messages

- *Specially packaged combination OCs (PREVEN) are available in the US for emergency contraception*

- *Effectiveness at preventing pregnancy is about 55% to 75%*

- *The most common side effects are nausea (50%) and vomiting (20%)*

- *Pretreatment with meclizine 50 mg significantly reduces nausea and vomiting associated with the Yuzpe method*

References

1. Food and Drug Administration Web site. FDA approves application for PREVEN emergency contraceptive kit. Available at: http://www.fda.gov/bbs/topics/ANSWERS/ANS00892.html. Accessed December 15, 1998.

2. Delbanco SF, Mauldon J, Smith MD. Little knowledge and limited practice: emergency contraceptive pills, the public, and the obstetrician-gynecologist. *Obstet Gynecol* 1997;89:1006-1011.

3. Trussell J, Rodriguez G, Ellertson C. New estimates of the effectiveness of the Yuzpe regimen of emergency contraception. *Contraception* 1998;57:363-369.

4. Creinin MD. A reassessment of efficacy of the Yuzpe regimen of emergency contraception. *Hum Reprod* 1997;12:101-103.

5. Task Force on Postovulatory Methods of Fertility Regulation. Randomised controlled trial of levonorgestrel versus the Yuzpe regimen of combined oral contraceptives for emergency contraception. *Lancet* 1998;352:428-433.

6. Glasier A. Emergency postcoital contraception. *N Engl J Med* 1997;337:1058-1064.

7. Food and Drug Administration. Prescription drug products: certain combined oral contraceptives for use as postcoital emergency contraception. *Federal Register* 1997;62:8610-8612.

8. Raymond EG, Creinin MD, Barnhart KT, et al. Meclizine for prevention of nausea associated with use of emergency contraceptive pills: a randomized trial. *Obstet Gynecol* 2000;95:271-277.

ii. Levonorgestrel Alone

A WHO-sponsored study has demonstrated that the progestin levonorgestrel, used alone, is a highly effective and well-tolerated form of emergency contraception.[1] The levonorgestrel regimen proved more effective than the Yuzpe method. On July 28, 1999, the FDA approved progestin-only emergency contraception. The product, Plan B™, contains two tablets of 0.75 mg levonorgestrel.

WHO Research

Early research indicated that progestin-only emergency contraception of levonorgestrel was as effective as the Yuzpe regimen, with significantly fewer side effects.[2] Prompted by these findings, WHO completed a larger Yuzpe vs levonorgestrel study.[1] Researchers conducted the double-blind, randomized trial in 21 centers worldwide, including Australia, Canada, China, India, New Zealand, Nigeria, Sweden, the United Kingdom, and the United States. Participants included women with regular menses not using hormonal contraception, who requested emergency contraception after unprotected intercourse occurring within the previous 72 hours. Follow-up data were available for 1,955 women.

Dosing

Approximately half of the women received an initial 0.75 mg levonorgestrel dose, followed by a second dose 12 hours later. The other half received the Yuzpe regimen. Nearly 50% of the women in each treatment group started treatment within 24 hours of unprotected intercourse. More than 80% did so within 48 hours.

Efficacy

Levonorgestrel alone was significantly better at preventing pregnancy. The relative risk of pregnancy in the levonorgestrel group was 0.4 (95% CI, 0.2-0.7), indicating a 60% lower likelihood of pregnancy compared to the Yuzpe regimen. Stated another way, the proportion of pregnancies prevented in the levonorgestrel group was 85% (compared with the predicted rate that would have occurred with no treatment). Using the same criteria, the Yuzpe method prevented only 57% of pregnancies.

Ellertson and colleagues questioned the superior efficacy of the levonorgestrel regimen.[3] Using the most up-to-date estimates of conception probabilities,[4] WHO still found the effectiveness of levonorgestrel to be 88%. As pointed out by WHO, the randomized, double-blind design eliminates many forms of bias. When WHO researchers used different methods to adjust for cycle day, other factors, and secondary analyses, levonorgestrel alone was consistently found to be more effective than the Yuzpe regimen.[5]

Figure 48

Effect of Delay of Treatment with Levonorgestrel or the Yuzpe Regimen on Pregnancy Rates

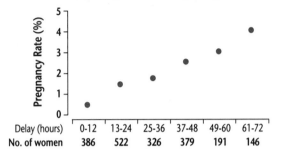

Delay (hours)	0-12	13-24	25-36	37-48	49-60	61-72
No. of women	386	522	326	379	191	146

Source: Piaggio G, von Hertzen H, Grimes DA, et al. Timing of emergency contraception with levonorgestrel or the Yuzpe regimen. Task Force on Postovulatory Methods of Fertility Regulation. Lancet 1999;353:721. Reproduced with permission of the copyright owner, The Lancet Ltd.

Timing of Treatment

Treatment efficacy, regardless of method, was greater the sooner the first dose was administered after sexual exposure. Analyses by WHO indicate that treatment with both regimens is most effective when given within 12 hours of unprotected sex (Figure 48). Comments published in letters to *The Lancet* questioned these results,[3,6] because an earlier analysis of nine published reports had suggested that treatment with the Yuzpe regimen had similar effectiveness whether given 1, 2, or 3 days after unprotected intercourse.[4]

Nonetheless, WHO found a consistent linear relationship between efficacy and the time from coitus to treatment.[7] Overall pregnancy rates increased from 0.5% (treatment within 12 hours) to 4.1% (treatment between 61 and 72 hours). The rising trend in pregnancy rates with increasing delay was significant ($p < 0.01$). Postponement of the first dose by 12 hours raised the odds of pregnancy by almost 50%.[5,7]

Side Effects

The levonorgestrel group had fewer side effects. With both regimens, the most commonly reported side effects were nausea and vomiting. Rates of nausea, however, were about 23% for the levonorgestrel group vs 51% for the Yuzpe group (p<0.01). Vomiting occurred in only 6% of the levonorgestrel group vs 19% for the Yuzpe group (p<0.01). As a result, significantly fewer women who received levonorgestrel alone required an extra dose due to vomiting.

The levonorgestrel-treated women also experienced significantly less dizziness and fatigue (p<0.01). Other undesirable effects associated with both methods were headache, breast tenderness, lower abdominal pain, diarrhea, and some irregular bleeding and spotting. In each category, the mean incidence of adverse events was lower in the levonorgestrel-only group.

Availability

The Plan B formulation has been used in other countries for 2 decades. A Hungarian company, Gedeon Richter, Ltd., manufactures the product for its North American distributor, Women's Capitol Corporation, a privately held company formed in 1997 to bring progestin-only emergency contraception to the US and Canadian markets.

Initial availability of Plan B has been limited. The product currently is available by prescription through Planned Parenthood clinics and clinicians registered with the Emergency Contraception Hotline (1-888-NOT-2-LATE) and the Emergency Contraception Web site (http://www.not-2-late.org). The product is also available at city, county, and state health departments; some hospitals; and college student health centers.

Take Home Messages

- *Levonorgestrel alone is a highly effective and well-tolerated form of emergency contraception*

- *Specially packaged levonorgestrel for emergency contraception is available in the US (Plan B)*

- *Data from WHO indicate levonorgestrel alone prevented 85% of pregnancies, while the combination regimen (Yuzpe method) prevented only 57% of pregnancies*

- *Efficacy of both the Yuzpe and progestin-only methods is greater the sooner the first dose is administered after sexual exposure*

Continued on next page

> **Take Home Messages** *(continued)*
>
> ■ *The rates of nausea and vomiting are significantly less among women using levonorgestrel compared to women using the combination regimen*

References

1. Task Force on Postovulatory Methods of Fertility Regulation. Randomised controlled trial of levonorgestrel versus the Yuzpe regimen of combined oral contraceptives for emergency contraception. *Lancet* 1998;352:428-433.

2. Ho PC, Kwan MSW. A prospective randomized comparison of levonorgestrel with the Yuzpe regimen in post-coital contraception. *Human Reprod* 1993;8: 389-392.

3. Ellertson C, Blanchard K, Webb A, et al. Emergency contraception. *Lancet* 1998;352:1477. Letter.

4. Trussell J, Ellertson C, Rodriguez G. The Yuzpe regimen of emergency contraception: how long after the morning after? *Obstet Gynecol* 1996;88: 150-154.

5. von Hertzen H, Piaggio G, Van Look PFA on behalf of the Task Force of Postovulatory Methods of Fertility Regulation. Emergency contraception with levonorgestrel or the Yuzpe regimen. *Lancet* 1998;352:1939. Letter.

6. Trussell J. Emergency contraception: WHO Task Force study. *Lancet* 1998; 352:1222-1223. Letter.

7. Piaggio G, von Hertzen H, Grimes DA, et al. Timing of emergency contraception with levonorgestrel or the Yuzpe regimen. Task Force on Postovulatory Methods of Fertility Regulation. *Lancet* 1999;353:721. Letter.

iii. Raising Awareness and Access

Despite the availability of two FDA-approved emergency contraceptive pills, patients are often unaware that emergency contraception exists. According to a 1997 telephone survey of 754 health care providers by the Kaiser Family Foundation, many clinicians only discuss emergency contraception when a patient takes the initiative to seek treatment, rather than talking about it as part of routine contraceptive counseling.[1] A companion survey of 1,000 women and 300 men aged 18 to 44 years found that many patients remain unaware or misinformed about emergency contraception and, thus, may not ask about it on their own. Once informed, nearly half of all women surveyed said they would consider emergency contraception if faced with the possibility of an unintended pregnancy.[2]

Clinicians need to counsel all reproductive age women and men about emergency contraception. Knowledge of and access to emergency contraception will only increase if clinicians feel more comfortable about prescribing the method and counsel their patients, particularly teens and young women, more consistently.[3] Another option to increase awareness is to suggest that young women also let their friends know about the method's availability.

Among women who have used emergency contraception, satisfaction is high.[4,5] A published report surveyed 235 women who used the Yuzpe regimen during a Kaiser Permanente demonstration project.[5] More than 90% of the women reported satisfaction with the method and nearly all (97%) said they would recommend emergency contraceptive pills to others. Only six participants reported dissatisfaction; five of these had become pregnant.

Resources are available to help increase awareness and incorporate emergency contraception into clinical practice (Table 27). In addition to the Emergency Contraception Hotline and Web site, a resource packet can provide clinicians with useful information and awareness tools. Available through Planned Parenthood for $5.00, the packet includes a resource manual for clinicians, a fact sheet, brochures for adults and adolescents, and a poster.

Because timing is of critical importance with emergency contraception,[6] clinicians should minimize access barriers. Prescribing by telephone is one way to improve timely access. By asking the patient three questions (Figure 49), clinicians can determine if an emergency contraception prescription is appropriate. If the response is "yes" to all three questions, the clinician may prescribe emergency contraception over the telephone. If one or more responses are negative, the patient may need a pregnancy test before emergency contraception can be prescribed.

Another approach to timely access is writing an advance prescription. For example, clinicians may want to give women a handout about emergency contraception and an advance prescription, especially if they are using condoms as their sole contraceptive method. The approach can help educate patients about emergency contraception and, if needed, help ensure that therapy is initiated as soon as possible after unprotected intercourse.

Results of a 1998 randomized controlled trial in the United Kingdom support advance prescription.[7] In the study, a group of 549 women self-administering emergency contraception via

Table 27

Resources for Providers and Patients

Emergency Contraception Hotline: 1-888-NOT-2-LATE (1-888-668-2528)

Established in February 1996 by the Reproductive Health Technologies Project and the Office of Population Research at Princeton University, this toll-free, automated, 24-hour telephone service provides information about emergency contraception in English and Spanish. The service also provides referrals to five health care providers in the caller's geographic area. Clinicians can join the hotline's referral network by completing an online form or by contacting the Emergency Contraception Hotline, 21 Prospect Ave., Princeton, NJ 08544.

Emergency Contraception Internet Site: http://www.not-2-late.org

Comprehensive information about emergency contraception —including answers to commonly asked questions—is available in English and Spanish on this Web site maintained by the Office of Population Research at Princeton University. The site describes available options for emergency contraception and provides photographs of each method. The site also includes a state-by-state directory of more than 2,000 US providers who prescribe emergency contraception.

Emergency Contraception Resource Packet

A comprehensive information packet, *Emergency Contraception: Resources for Providers*, is available to clinicians through Planned Parenthood Federation of America (PPFA). Jointly sponsored by ACOG and the Association of Reproductive Health Professionals and developed with support from the Henry J. Kaiser Family Foundation, the packet includes the following materials:

- *Emergency Contraception: A Resource Manual for Providers*
- "Facts About Emergency Contraception" (four-page fact sheet)
- "Emergency Contraception: What You Need to Know" (adult patient brochure)
- "Just Had Sex?" (teen patient brochure)
- "ECP Instructions for Use" (insert)
- "Just Had Sex?" (8" x 10" poster)
- *ACOG Practice Patterns*, December 1996 (emergency contraception practice guidelines)

To order the entire packet ($5.00 each) or bulk copies of individual pieces, contact the PPFA Marketing Department at 810 Seventh Avenue, New York, NY 10019 or call 1-800-669-0156.

advance prescription had lower rates of unintended pregnancy than 522 controls who had to visit a clinician to obtain emergency contraceptive pills. Women with advance prescription were no more likely to use emergency contraception repeatedly and their use of other contraceptive methods was no different from that of women in the control group.[7]

Pharmacist Dispensing

Pharmacists can increase access to emergency contraception.[8] A pilot program in Washington state, which used collaborative prescribing agreements between clinicians and pharmacists, found that allowing pharmacists to dispense emergency contraception under established protocols increased its use. A media campaign informed women about the availability of emergency contraception through local pharmacies. The pharmacist-dispensing program dramatically increased the use of emergency contraception. In the program's first 4 months, pharmacists dispensed almost 2,800 prescriptions for emergency contraception.[8] These favorable results have encouraged other states to consider implementing similar programs.

Figure 49

Telephone Prescribing: Three Questions to Ask

Important questions to ask a patient calling to request emergency contraception:

1. **Have you had unprotected sex or a problem with your birth control (such as condom breakage) during the last 3 days?**

    Date _____

2. **Did your last menstrual period begin less than 4 weeks ago?**

    Date _____

3. **Was the timing and duration of your last menstrual period normal?**

If the patient responds "yes" to all three questions, a clinician may prescribe emergency contraception over the telephone.

Adapted from ACOG, *Emergency Contraception: A Resource Manual for Providers*, 1998.

Counseling Suggestions

When a patient is in need of emergency contraception, appropriate counseling is an important part of therapy. Clinicians may wish to follow these suggestions:

- *Ensure that the patient does not want to become pregnant.*

- *Describe how to use emergency contraception correctly.*

- *Provide written instructions.*

- *Inform her of potential side effects (eg, nausea, vomiting, cramping).*

- *Point out that emergency contraception provides no protection against (or treatment for) sexually transmitted disease.*

- *Stress that the method is for "emergency" use only. Remind patients that regular use of a primary contraceptive method (with emergency contraceptive use only when needed) is more effective than using no primary method followed by emergency contraception after unprotected intercourse.*

- *For women using some form of birth control, remind the patient to use ongoing contraception immediately because ovulation may be delayed, but is not prevented. For women not using birth control, the "close call" experience may be a good opportunity for clinicians to reinforce the importance of consistent use of a reliable contraceptive method.*

- *Inform the patient that her period may arrive a few days earlier or later than normal.*

- *Explain that emergency contraception can fail. Suggest that the patient return for a pregnancy test (or that she administer a home pregnancy test) if her period does not resume within 3 weeks.*

- *Encourage the patient to call if any questions arise.*

Take Home Messages

- *Adolescent and adult women may not be aware of emergency contraception*

- *Surveys indicate that women who have used emergency contraception are highly satisfied with the method*

- *Resources are available from ACOG and Planned Parenthood to help clinicians increase awareness and incorporate emergency contraception into their practice*

- *Clinicians may want to consider giving patients an advance prescription*

References

1. 1997 Kaiser Family Foundation Survey of Health Care Providers on Emergency Contraception. Fact Finders, Inc.: December 18, 1997 (press release).

2. 1997 Kaiser Family Foundation Survey of Americans on Emergency Contraception. Princeton Survey Research Associates: December 18, 1997 (press release).

3. Schein AB. Pregnancy prevention using emergency contraception: efficacy, attitudes, and limitations to use. *J Pediatr Adolesc Gynecol* 1999;12:3-9.

4. Breitbart V, Castle MA, Walsh K, et al. The impact of patient experience on practice: the acceptability of emergency contraceptive pills in inner-city clinics. *J Am Med Womens Assoc* 1998;53(suppl 2):255-257,265.

5. Harvey SM, Beckman LJ, Sherman C, et al. Women's experience and satisfaction with emergency contraception. *Fam Plann Perspect* 1999;31: 237-240, 260.

6. Piaggio G, von Hertzen H, Grimes DA, et al. Timing of emergency contraception with levonorgestrel or the Yuzpe regimen. Task Force on Postovulatory Methods of Fertility Regulation. *Lancet* 1999;353:721. Letter.

7. Glasier A, Baird D. The effects of self-administering emergency contraception. *N Engl J Med* 1998;339:1-4.

8. Wells ES, Hutchings J, Gardner JS, et al. Using pharmacies in Washington state to expand access to emergency contraception. *Fam Plann Perspect* 1998;30:288-290.

4.4: Progestin-Only OCs

Progestin-only oral contraceptives, sometimes called the "minipill," are not widely used in the United States. Fewer than 1% of US oral contraceptive prescriptions are for progestin-only pills.[1] Their use tends to be concentrated in select populations, most notably breastfeeding women and those with contraindications to the estrogen in combined OCs.

Two formulations of progestin-only pills (POPs) are available in the US. One contains 75 μg norgestrel; the other has 350 μg norethindrone. The dosage in both formulations has remained relatively constant since their introduction in the mid-1970s. POPs have a lower dose of progestin than do combined OCs. (Low-dose combined OCs typically contain 200 to 300 μg norgestrel or 400 to 1,000 μg norethindrone.)

Mechanisms of Action

Progestin-only oral contraceptives prevent conception through a combination of mechanisms (Figure 50). Investigators have identified four potential modes of action for POPs:

1. *Suppression of ovulation:* POPs have a dampening effect on the midcycle peaks of luteinizing hormone (LH) and follicle-stimulating hormone (FSH), although effects on basal levels are more variable.[2,3] Unlike combined OCs, POPs do not uniformly suppress ovulation in all cycles.[4,5] Moreover, the extent of ovarian response varies widely among individual POP users and is an unreliable mechanism for preventing pregnancy.[6] In general, POPs are believed to suppress ovulation in about half of cycles.[1]

2. *Alteration of cervical mucus:* POPs reduce cervical mucus volume, increase its viscosity, and alter its molecular structure. The result is a "hostile" or "blocked" cervical mucus that decreases the possibility of sperm penetration.[7]

3. *Alteration of the endometrium:* POPs may interfere with the cyclic development of the uterine lining, making it unsuitable for ovum implantation. POP progestins appear to reduce the number and size of endometrial glands and inhibit the synthesis of progesterone receptors in the endometrium.[8]

4. *Alteration of the fallopian tubes:* POPs may affect cilia in the fallopian tubes, decreasing the intensity and frequency of their action. The result may be a slowing effect on the rate of ovum transport.[2]

Figure 50

Potential Mechanisms of Action of Progestin-Only Oral Contraceptives

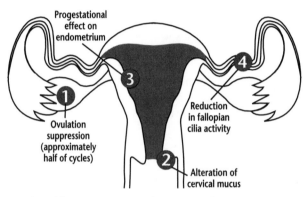

Source: Adapted from McCann MF, et al, 1994 (see reference 1).

Efficacy and Dosing Schedule

Failure rates during typical use are difficult to compute for POPs because surveys often do not differentiate between combined and progestin-only OCs. Although some estimates place the failure rate of POPs at 5%,[1] because compliance has the most impact on effectiveness, the typical failure rate for POPs probably is similar to those for combined OCs—about 7% during the first 12 months.[9] This rate is substantially lower than the typical use failure rates of other immediately reversible contraceptive methods, such as the male condom and diaphragm (both 14%).[9]

Efficacy of progestin-only pills requires consistent administration. Serum progestin levels in POP users peak about 2 hours after administration.[1] Rapid distribution and elimination bring serum levels back to near baseline within 24 hours. The POP's protection starts to diminish after 20 hours, so if each pill is not taken within

24 hours of the previous one, the risk of contraceptive failure goes up substantially. Consequently, POP users should take their pills at the same time every day. Variation of even a few hours can place POP users at risk of unintended pregnancy.

Provided the POP is taken at the same time every day without interruption, the time of day is not crucial. However, the cervical mucus effect—considered to be one of the key mechanisms of action—is believed to peak about 4 hours after ingestion and remain present for 16 to 19 hours.[1] Consequently, taking the pill at bedtime theoretically could reduce contraceptive efficacy, assuming that bedtime is the most likely time of intercourse. Some investigators have dubbed POPs the "teatime" pill, recommending they be taken in the late afternoon or early evening for maximum efficacy at bedtime.[1] Optimum pill-taking schedules may differ for teenagers, however. Clinicians should consider asking teen POP users about their most likely time of intercourse to help guide pill-taking recommendations.

POP users should be prepared to use a backup method of contraception in the event of late or missed pills. In the case of POPs, a late pill is generally considered one that is taken more than 3 hours after the established daily time of administration. If a pill is forgotten, it should be taken as soon as it is remembered; the next pill should then be taken at the regular time. Backup contraception should be used for 48 hours.[1] Although some have advocated using additional protection for up to 7 days, this recommendation appears to be based on a desire to make the backup instructions uniform across POPs and combined OCs. However, because of the rapid resumption of the cervical mucus effect, 48 hours of additional contraception should provide sufficient protection in the event of missed POPs.[1] Clinicians also should inform POP users of the availability of emergency contraception.

Starting POP Use

- If progestin-only OCs are begun within the first 5 days of the menstrual cycle, the woman does not need to use a backup method of contraception.

- If progestin-only OCs are begun after day 5 of menses, the woman should use a backup contraceptive for 48 hours until the contraceptive effect on the cervical mucus peaks.

- POPs may be initiated immediately after an abortion.

Side Effects and Risks

Menstrual Cycle

The primary side effect of progestin-only pills is menstrual cycle disruption. Less common side effects include headache, breast tenderness, nausea, and dizziness. POP users commonly have spotting or breakthrough bleeding, amenorrhea, or shortened cycles. The variability of menstrual cycle lengths can be especially troubling for users. Menstrual side effects are the most frequently cited reason for method-related discontinuation of POPs.

A 1982 randomized, double-blind trial by WHO evaluated menstrual effects in 258 POP users. During the first 3 months of use, an average of 53% of users reported frequent bleeding, 22% reported prolonged bleeding, 13% reported irregular bleeding, and 6% reported amenorrhea (Figure 51). Although frequency of these effects decreased by cycle 12, one-quarter of POP users in the study discontinued because of bleeding disturbances.[10]

Ectopic Pregnancy

Overall, POP use protects against ectopic pregnancy by lowering the chance of conception. If POP users get pregnant, an average of

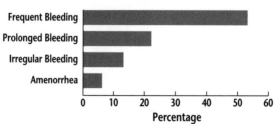

Figure 51

Percentage of Progestin-Only Pill Users Reporting Menstrual Effects During First 3 Months of Use

Source: World Health Organization, 1982 (see reference 10).

6% to 10% of pregnancies will be extrauterine—substantially higher than the proportion of ectopic pregnancies among noncontracepting women (about 2%).[1] However, if 7% of POP users become pregnant during typical use and 10% of these pregnancies are extrauterine, the overall risk of ectopic pregnancy among POP users is 0.7%—one-third that of the general population.

Women with a history of ectopic pregnancy may use POPs; however, all women should be alert to symptoms of ectopic pregnancy, including abdominal or pelvic discomfort and amenorrhea.

Cardiovascular Safety

POPs do not appear to increase the risk of cardiovascular disease. A 1998 WHO case-control study found no significant increase in the risk of stroke (RR=1.1; 95% CI, 0.6-1.9), venous thromboembolism (RR=1.8; 95% CI, 0.8-4.2), or acute myocardial infarction (RR=1.0; 95% CI, 0.2-6.0) among users of progestin-only pills (Figure 52).[11]

POPs also appear to have little or no effect on lipid metabolism, carbohydrate metabolism, coagulation factors, or hypertension.

Figure 52

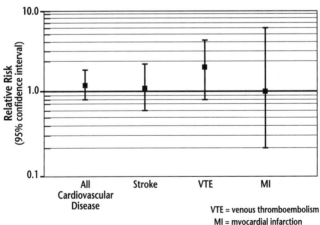

Risk of Cardiovascular Disease among Users of Progestin-Only Oral Contraceptives by Disease Type

VTE = venous thromboembolism
MI = myocardial infarction

Source: World Health Organization, 1998 (see reference 11).

POPs may be particularly appropriate for women who are hypertensive, at increased risk of thrombosis, experience migraine (vascular) headaches, or are cigarette smokers over age 35 years.[1]

Cancer

Few data are available regarding progestin-only pills and cancer. No evidence exists concerning whether POPs protect against endometrial or ovarian cancers. Similarly, little is known about the risk of cervical cancer or breast cancer among users of POPs. Scant available data do not suggest an elevated risk.[1]

Type 2 Diabetes Mellitus

A 1998 study reported an increased risk of type 2 diabetes mellitus in breastfeeding Latina POP users with prior gestational diabetes.[12] Of the 900 postpartum Latina women in the study, 78 used a progestin-only OC while breastfeeding. After adjustment for potential confounding factors, POP use increased the risk of diabetes mellitus nearly threefold compared with equivalent use of low-dose combination OCs (RR=2.9; 95% CI, 1.6-5.3). Risk magnitude increased with duration of use. Investigators found no increase in risk among study participants who used combination OCs or nonhormonal contraceptive methods. The authors suggested that POPs should be prescribed with caution in breastfeeding Latina women with recent gestational diabetes mellitus, if at all; however, more evidence is needed to confirm these results.

WHO Prescribing Guidelines

The World Health Organization lists few conditions under which POP use is not recommended (Table 28).[13] Generally considered very conservative, the WHO guidelines list only one absolute contraindication to initiating POP use—pregnancy. The remaining conditions fall under WHO's Category 3, the designation assigned when the theoretical or proven risks usually outweigh the advantages of using a contraceptive method. In Category 3 cases, patients should only use the method if the clinician judges that the benefits outweigh the risks.

Table 28

WHO Guidelines: Conditions Under Which Starting Progestin-Only OCs May Not Be Recommended

WHO Category 3*

— Unexplained abnormal vaginal bleeding

— Current or past breast cancer[†]

— Active viral hepatitis[†]

— Severe (decompensated) cirrhosis of the liver

— Benign or malignant liver tumors

— Schistosomiasis with severe fibrosis of the liver

— Use of enzyme-inducing antibiotics (rifampin and griseofulvin)

— Use of enzyme-inducing anticonvulsants

— Breastfeeding, less than 6 weeks postpartum[§]

WHO Category 4**

— Pregnancy

* Category 3: use of method not usually recommended unless other, more appropriate methods are not available or not acceptable.

** Category 4: method not to be used.

† WHO recommendations are based on theoretical concerns, but no data are available.

§ WHO recommendations apply to women exclusively breastfeeding. Breastfeeding women supplementing with formula should begin POPs 3 weeks postpartum.

Source: World Health Organization, 1996 (see reference 13).

Breastfeeding Women

Progestin-only pills may be particularly suited for use in breast-feeding women who desire hormonal contraception. The World Health Organization and other organizations advocate the use of POPs over combined OCs in breastfeeding women. POPs have no adverse effect on breastfeeding performance and may enhance lactation by stimulating greater prolactin release, similar to the effect seen with DMPA.[14]

Data from *high-dose* combined OCs indicated a negative impact on breast milk quality and quantity and a greater likelihood of infant exposure to contraceptive hormones.[15] Importantly, however, low-dose combination OCs have not been shown to have any adverse effects on milk production or breastfeeding. (For further discussion, see the section on use of combination OCs in breastfeeding women.)

The timing of POP initiation in breastfeeding women is a subject of debate. In general, women who are exclusively breastfeeding may begin using POPs 6 weeks after giving birth.[13] Breastfeeding women who are giving formula supplements to their babies and nonbreastfeeding women should start POPs 3 weeks postpartum because of decreased suppression of ovulation.[1]

Take Home Messages

- Typical use failure rates for POPs are similar to those for combined OCs (7% in the first 12 months)

- POP effectiveness depends upon consistent use at the same time each day

- POPs lack estrogen-related risks and side effects; however, they also lack some of the benefits, including menstrual cycle regularity, acne improvement, and potential use in treating certain medical conditions

- The estimated overall risk of ectopic pregnancy among POP users is 0.7%—one-third that of the general population

---

References

1. McCann MF, Potter LS. Progestin-only oral contraception: a comprehensive review. *Contraception* 1994;50(suppl 1):S9-S195.

2. Landgren BM, Balogh A, Shin MW, et al. Hormonal effects of the 300 μg norethisterone (NET) minipill. 2. Daily gonadotropin levels in 43 subjects during a pretreatment cycle and during the second month of NET administration. *Contraception* 1979;20:585-605.

3. Landgren BM, Lager S, Diczfalusy E. Hormonal effects of the 300 μg norethisterone (NET) minipill. 3. Comparison of the short-term (2nd month) and medium-term (6th month) effects on 21 subjects. *Contraception* 1981;23:269-299.

4. Oberti C, Dabancens A, Garcia-Huidobro M, et al. Low dosage oral progestogens to control fertility. II. Morphologic modifications in the gonad and oviduct. *Obstet Gynecol* 1974;43:285-294.

5. Tayob Y, Adams J, Jacobs HS, et al. Ultrasound demonstration of increased frequency of functional ovarian cysts in women using progestogen-only oral contraception. *Br J Obstet Gynaecol* 1985;92:1003-1009.

6. Landgren BM, Diczfalusy E. Hormonal effects of the 300 µg norethisterone (NET) minipill. 1. Daily steroid levels in 43 subjects during a pretreatment cycle and during the second month of NET administration. *Contraception* 1980;21:87-113.

7. Martinez-Manautou J, Giner-Velasquez J, Cortes-Gallegos V, et al. Daily progestogen for contraception: a clinical study. *BMJ* 1967;2:730-732.

8. Kim-Bjorklund T, Landgren BM, Johannisson E. Morphometric studies of the endometrium, the fallopian tube and the corpus luteum during contraception with the 300 µg norethisterone (NET) minipill. *Contraception* 1991;43: 459-474.

9. Fu H, Darroch JE, Haas T, et al. Contraceptive failure rates: new estimates from the 1995 National Survey of Family Growth. *Fam Plann Perspect* 1999;31:58-63.

10. WHO Task Force on Oral Contraceptives. A randomized, double-blind study of two combined and two progestogen-only oral contraceptives. *Contraception* 1982;25:243-252.

11. WHO Collaborative Study of Cardiovascular Disease and Steroid Contraception. Cardiovascular disease and use of oral and injectable progestogen-only contraceptives and combined injectable contraceptives: results of an international, multicenter, case-control study. *Contraception* 1998;57:315-324.

12. Kjos SL, Peters RK, Xiang A, et al. Contraception and the risk of type 2 diabetes mellitus in Latina women with prior gestational diabetes mellitus. *JAMA* 1998;280:533-538.

13. Family Planning Programme. *Improving Access to Quality Care in Family Planning. Medical Eligibility Criteria for Contraceptive Use.* Geneva: World Health Organization; 1996:53-68.

14. Fraser IS. A review of the use of progestogen-only minipills for contraception during lactation. *Reprod Fertil Dev* 1991;3:245-254.

15. WHO Task Force on Oral Contraceptives. Effects of hormonal contraceptives on milk volume and infant growth. *Contraception* 1984;30:505-522.

Appendix A: Laboratory Values

Test	Effect on Values	Comment
T_4 thyroxine (total T_4)	Increase	Estrogens increase hepatic synthesis of TBG in a dose-related fashion, increasing TBG and related proteins. TBG and related tests return to normal about 2 months after OC discontinuation.
Thyroxine-binding globulin (TBG)	Increase	
Triiodothyronine resin uptake (T_3 uptake)	Decrease	
Free T_3, reverse T_3, thyroid-stimulating hormone (TSH)	No effect	
Free T_4	No effect or increase	
Cortisol-binding globulin (CBG)	Increase	Can effect lab testing for Cushing syndrome.
Free cortisol	No effect or modest increase	
Sex hormone-binding globulin (SHBG)	Increase	
Free testosterone	Decrease	
Total cholesterol	Increase	In general, estrogens ↑HDL and ↓LDL. Progestins ↓HDL, especially HDL$_2$, ↑LDL, and ↓TG and ↓VLDL.* Although combination OCs can alter lipoproteins, no long-term adverse effect on heart disease has been shown.
HDL* cholesterol	May increase or decrease	
LDL* cholesterol	Increase or no effect	
Triglycerides (TG)	No effect or increase	
Erythrocyte sedimentation rate	No effect or may increase or decrease	
Total iron-binding capacity	Increase	
Serum transferrin	Increase	

*HDL=high-density lipoprotein, LDL=low-density lipoprotein, VLDL=very low-density lipoprotein.

Source: Adapted from Goldzieher JW, Fotherby K, eds. Pharmacology of the Contraceptive Steroids. New York: Raven Press; 1994.

Appendix B: Low-Dose OCs Available in Canada

Appendix B provides, in alphabetical order, the name, steroid content, and manufacturer of OCs currently on the Canadian market. The table also further subdivides OCs into monophasic, multiphasic, and progestin-only preparations and identifies the OC by the type of progestin—either gonane or estrane.

Low-Dose Oral Contraceptives Available in Canada

Product Name*	Manufacturer	Estrogen	µg	Progestin	mg
Monophasic preparations					
20 µg estrogen					
Gonane progestin					
Alesse	Wyeth-Ayerst Canada Inc.	EE	20	Levonorgestrel	0.10
Estrane progestin					
Minestrin 1/20	Parke-Davis	EE	20	Norethindrone acetate	1.00
30-35 µg estrogen					
Gonane progestin					
Cyclen	Janssen-Ortho Inc.	EE	35	Norgestimate	0.25
Marvelon	Organon Canada Inc.	EE	30	Desogestrel	0.15
Min-Ovral	Wyeth-Ayerst Canada Inc.	EE	30	Levonorgestrel	0.15
Ortho-Cept	Janssen-Ortho Inc.	EE	30	Desogestrel	0.15
Estrane progestin					
Brevicon 0.5/35	Searle Canada Inc.	EE	35	Norethindrone	0.50
Brevicon 1/35	Searle Canada Inc.	EE	35	Norethindrone	1.00
Demulen 30	Searle Canada Inc.	EE	30	Ethynodiol diacetate	2.00
Loestrin 1.5/30	Parke-Davis	EE	30	Norethindrone acetate	1.50
Ortho-0.5/35	Janssen-Ortho Inc.	EE	35	Norethindrone	0.50
Ortho-1/35	Janssen-Ortho Inc.	EE	35	Norethindrone	1.00
Select 1/35	Searle Canada Inc.	EE	35	Norethindrone	1.00

Multiphasic preparations

Gonane progestin

Product Name*	Manufacturer	Estrogen	µg	Progestin	mg
Tri-Cyclen	Janssen-Ortho Inc.	EE	35 (21)**	Norgestimate	0.18 (7)
				Norgestimate	0.215 (7)
				Norgestimate	0.25 (7)
Triphasil	Wyeth-Ayerst Canada Inc.	EE	30 (6)	Levonorgestrel	0.05 (6)
		EE	40 (5)	Levonorgestrel	0.075 (5)
		EE	30 (10)	Levonorgestrel	0.125 (10)
Triquilar	Berlex Canada Inc.	EE	30 (6)	Levonorgestrel	0.05 (6)
		EE	40 (5)	Levonorgestrel	0.075 (5)
		EE	30 (10)	Levonorgestrel	0.125 (10)

Estrane progestin

Product Name*	Manufacturer	Estrogen	µg	Progestin	mg
Ortho-10/11	Janssen-Ortho Inc.	EE	35 (21)	Norethindrone	0.50 (10)
				Norethindrone	1.00 (11)
Ortho-7/7/7	Janssen-Ortho Inc.	EE	35 (21)	Norethindrone	0.50 (7)
				Norethindrone	0.75 (7)
				Norethindrone	1.00 (7)
Synphasic	Searle Canada Inc.	EE	35 (21)	Norethindrone	0.50 (7)
				Norethindrone	1.00 (9)
				Norethindrone	0.50 (5)

Progestin only

Estrane progestin

Product Name*	Manufacturer	Estrogen	µg	Progestin	mg
Micronor	Janssen-Ortho Inc.	None		Norethindrone	0.35

EE = ethinyl estradiol
* Product names are for identification purposes only and do not imply endorsement.
** ( ) = number of days each dosage is taken.

Appendix C: List of Abbreviations

ACOG	American College of Obstetricians and Gynecologists
AIDS	Acquired immunodeficiency syndrome
CASH	Cancer and Steroid Hormone Study
CDC	Centers for Disease Control and Prevention
DMPA	Depot medroxyprogesterone acetate
EE	Ethinyl estradiol
FDA	Food and Drug Administration
FPA	Family Planning Association
FSH	Follicle-stimulating hormone
HBV	Hepatitis B virus
HIV	Human immunodeficiency virus
HMO	Health maintenance organization
HPV	Human papillomavirus
IUD	Intrauterine device
LH	Luteinizing hormone
MI	Myocardial infarction
NIH	National Institutes of Health
NSFG	National Survey of Family Growth
OC	Oral contraceptive
OR	Odds ratio
PID	Pelvic inflammatory disease
PMS	Premenstrual syndrome
POP	Progestin-only pill
RBA	Relative binding affinity
RCGP	Royal College of General Practitioners
RR	Relative risk
SHBG	Sex hormone-binding globulin
STD	Sexually transmitted disease
UK	United Kingdom
US	United States
VTE	Venous thromboembolism
WHO	World Health Organization

Index

CME Quiz Questions

Section 1 Quiz

1. Which of the following was a contaminant in early birth control pill formulations that later was found to contribute to cycle control and efficacy
   a. ethinyl estradiol
   b. norethynodrel
   c. mestranol
   d. norethindrone

2. According to the National Survey of Family Growth, between 1982 and 1995, among women aged 35-39 years, use of oral contraceptives
   a. remained stable
   b. doubled
   c. dropped by 25%
   d. dropped by 50%

3. According to data from IMS Health, approximately what percentage of 1998 retail OC prescriptions were written for low-dose pills (≤ 35 µg ethinyl estradiol)
   a. 58%
   b. 68%
   c. 90%
   d. 99%

4. All of the following contribute to the efficacy of combination oral contraceptives containing low doses of estrogen, EXCEPT
   a. synergistic pituitary inhibition by ethinyl estrogen and a progestin
   b. progestin pharmacokinetics
   c. progestin's effect on the cervical mucus
   d. individual differences in steroid metabolism

5. Among OC progestins available in the US, which has the highest posthepatic bioavailability
   a. norethindrone
   b. levonorgestrel
   c. desogestrel
   d. norgestimate

6. All of the following are reasons why oral contraceptives are generally beneficial for acne, EXCEPT
   a. OCs lower sex hormone-binding globulin levels
   b. OCs suppress androgen production from the ovary
   c. OCs suppress androgen production from the adrenal gland
   d. OCs reduce free testosterone levels

7. The primary goal of the World Health Organization and other international organizations when revising medical eligibility criteria for contraception was to
   a. evaluate barrier methods to prevent sexually transmitted disease
   b. increase the number of methods available
   c. improve access to contraception without causing undue risk to patients
   d. review cancer data on hormonal methods

8. The World Health Organization's revised medical eligibility criteria list all of the following conditions as a Category 1, requiring no restriction of OC use, EXCEPT
   a. thyroid disease
   b. trophoblastic disease
   c. family history of breast cancer
   d. mild hypertension

9. Which of the following screening measures is necessary before prescribing combination OCs
   a. blood pressure measurement
   b. lipid profile
   c. glucose tolerance test
   d. urinalysis

10. All of the following factors influence the occurrence of breakthrough bleeding with OC use, EXCEPT
    a. cigarette smoking
    b. chlamydial infection
    c. age
    d. missed pills

Section 2 Quiz

11. The Nurses' Health Study found that use of OCs has what effect on the risk of developing type 2 (non-insulin-dependent) diabetes
    a. decreases risk by 25%
    b. does not increase risk
    c. increases risk by 35%
    d. increases risk by 55%

12. Data from the Kaiser Permanente HMO in the United States indicate that low-dose OC users, compared to nonusers, have what risk of all types of stroke
    a. 40% increased risk
    b. 35% increased risk
    c. about the same risk
    d. 20% decreased risk

13. Data from WHO and the Royal College of General Practitioners suggest the risk of myocardial infarction among women taking OCs is
    a. increased by about 45%
    b. increased by about 30% for past users
    c. not increased among nonsmoking women
    d. decreased by about 25% for past users

14. The factor V Leiden mutation is present in what percentage of asymptomatic Caucasian women
    a. fewer than 5%
    b. approximately 10%
    c. approximately 20%
    d. more than 30%

15. According to a recent report based on a WHO scientific group meeting, each of the following potential biases or objections to the VTE research on "third-generation" OCs can be answered, EXCEPT
    a. selective prescribing
    b. attrition of susceptibles
    c. preferential diagnosis
    d. the 20 µg paradox

16. The Collaborative Group on Hormonal Factors in Breast Cancer found that among OC users, the slightly elevated risk of having breast cancer diagnosed disappeared how many years after stopping OC use
    a. 5 years
    b. 10 years
    c. 15 years
    d. 20 years

17. In the United States, during 1962-1988, mortality rates from primary liver cancer and other primary liver neoplasms have
    a. decreased by 10% among women and men
    b. decreased by 10% among women only
    c. remained stable among women and increased among men
    d. doubled among men

18. The 1994 analysis of the Oxford Family Planning Association Oral Contraception Study found what relationship between OCs and the risk of benign gallbladder disease
    a. no relationship
    b. 30% increased risk
    c. 40% increased risk
    d. 30% increased risk among nulliparous women

19. The World Health Organization's revised medical eligibility criteria suggest that among women with sickle cell anemia
    a. OCs present no risks to the patient
    b. the benefits of OCs generally outweigh the risks
    c. the risks of OCs generally outweigh the benefits
    d. OCs should not be used

20. The World Health Organization recommends that women not use combination OCs if they have which of the following types of headache
    a. cluster headache
    b. tension headache
    c. migraine without aura
    d. migraine with aura

Section 3 Quiz

21. Which of the following noncontraceptive health benefits of OCs has been shown in at least one study to encourage consistent pill use among adolescents
    a. relief of dysmenorrhea
    b. reduced risk of ovarian cancer
    c. decreased risk of benign breast disease
    d. decreased risk of anemia

22. The Cancer and Steroid Hormone Study found women who had ever taken oral contraceptives had an average decrease in the risk of ovarian cancer of
    a. 10%
    b. 40%
    c. 70%
    d. 90%

23. Overall, OCs reduce the risk of endometrial cancer by about how much
    a. 20%
    b. 40%
    c. 50%
    d. 80%

24. Recent data from the Nurses' Health Study found a significant protective effect of OCs against colorectal cancer after how many months of OC use
    a. 12
    b. 24
    c. 48
    d. 96

25. Prescribing a drug for an indication other than those included in FDA-approved labeling
    a. is proper if based on rational scientific theory or reliable medical opinion
    b. is illegal
    c. is subject to limitations set forth in the Food, Drug and Cosmetic Act
    d. must be based on evidence from randomized controlled trials

26. Considerable evidence supports each of the following uses of combined OCs, EXCEPT
    a. treatment of acne
    b. hastening the regression of existing ovarian cysts
    c. relief of dysmenorrhea
    d. treatment of hirsutism

27. The 1994 ACOG/Gallup poll found that about what percentage of women thought there were no other health benefits of the pill other than pregnancy prevention
    a. 15%
    b. 20%
    c. 40%
    d. 50%

28. In a survey of faculty, students, and employees of Yale University, about what percentage of women reported that they believed the pill causes breast cancer
    a. one-tenth
    b. one-quarter
    c. one-third
    d. one-half

29. According to a European survey of about 6,700 OC users by Rosenberg et al, those who experience two side effects are how much more likely to discontinue than users who experience no side effects
   a. 1.5 times as likely
   b. twice as likely
   c. three times as likely
   d. four times as likely

30. According to an analysis of 1995 NSFG data, approximately what proportion of OC discontinuers are using no method of contraception 3 months later
   a. one-tenth
   b. one-fifth
   c. one-quarter
   d. one-half

Section 4 Quiz

31. Emans et al found that an overwhelming majority of teens seen in a suburban private practice were concerned with what potential side effect of oral contraceptives
   a. acne
   b. infertility
   c. weight gain
   d. blood clots

32. A survey of high school students in Massachusetts found that teens who knew their doctors provided confidential care were about how many times more likely to discuss sexuality-related issues than teens who didn't believe their care was confidential
   a. no more likely
   b. two times more likely
   c. three times more likely
   d. four times more likely

33. What is the association between hormonal contraception use and HIV susceptibility
    a. hormonal contraception use doubles HIV risk
    b. hormonal contraception use reduces HIV risk by half
    c. hormonal contraception use does not affect HIV risk
    d. studies are conflicting and data are inconclusive

34. According to a 1998 study by the World Health Organization, levonorgestrel-only emergency contraception prevented what proportion of pregnancies that would have occurred without treatment
    a. 85%
    b. 75%
    c. 65%
    d. 55%

35. In the 1998 WHO trial of emergency contraception, women using the traditional Yuzpe method had about how much vomiting compared to those using levonorgestrel alone
    a. one-quarter less
    b. two-thirds less
    c. twice as much
    d. three times as much

36. Progestin-only and combination OCs used as emergency contraception are most effective when administered within how many hours after unprotected intercourse
    a. ≤12
    b. 24
    c. 48
    d. 72

37. The estimated first-year "typical use" failure rate for progestin-only OCs is
    a. 3%
    b. 7%
    c. 12%
    d. 18%

38. A progestin-only pill is considered "late" if it is taken more than how many hours after the established daily time of administration
    a. 1 hour
    b. 3 hours
    c. 6 hours
    d. 12 hours

39. If a progestin-only pill is taken late or missed, backup contraception should be used for at least
    a. 48 hours
    b. 96 hours
    c. 7 days
    d. 14 days

40. With regard to pharmacology and dosing schedule for progestin-only OCs, each of the following is true, EXCEPT
    a. serum progestin levels peak about 2 hours after administration
    b. the cervical mucus effect peaks about 4 hours after administration
    c. the ideal time of ingestion for most users is bedtime
    d. dosing schedule variation of a few hours increases risk of unintended pregnancy

CME Quiz Answer Form — Section 1

Modern Oral Contraception

After you have circled your answers to the questions, complete the information below and on the reverse side. This form must be filled out completely in order for you to receive proper credit. Please print clearly. Enclose a check for $15.00 payable to Dannemiller Memorial Educational Foundation. Mail to the address shown below. The Post Office will not deliver without proper postage.

Expiration Date: This credit is valid through June 30, 2001. No credit will be given after this date.

Dannemiller Memorial Educational Foundation
Attn: Contraception Report/99-40e
12500 Network Blvd., Suite 101, San Antonio, TX 78249-3302

Name _____ Degree _____

Street _____

City _____ State _____

Zip Code _____ Phone _____

Nursing License Number/State _____

Actual amount of time spent in this activity was: _____ hours _____ minutes.
(If blank, the Dannemiller Foundation assumes the participant spent 2 hours studying this material.)

Record your answers by circling the appropriate letter for each question.

1. a b c d   6. a b c d
2. a b c d   7. a b c d
3. a b c d   8. a b c d
4. a b c d   9. a b c d
5. a b c d   10. a b c d

80% (8 correct answers) constitutes a passing grade.

Please cut this page out and send to Dannemiller with your CME fee.

Evaluation Questionnaire

Modern Oral Contraception, Section 1

1. Please rate this program with respect to:

Overall quality of material:	☐ Excellent	☐ Very Good	☐ Good	☐ Fair	☐ Poor
Content of the section:	☐ Excellent	☐ Very Good	☐ Good	☐ Fair	☐ Poor
Usefulness in your practice:	☐ Excellent	☐ Very Good	☐ Good	☐ Fair	☐ Poor
How well course objectives were met:	☐ Excellent	☐ Very Good	☐ Good	☐ Fair	☐ Poor

2. Was there commercial or promotional bias in the presentation? ☐ Yes   ☐ No

   If yes, please explain: _____

3. Additional comments: _____

   _____

   _____

Your e-mail address: _____

May Dannemiller contact you regarding CME program outcomes?   ☐ Yes   ☐ No

Modern Oral Contraception

CME Quiz Answer Form

Section 2

After you have circled your answers to the questions, complete the information below and on the reverse side. This form must be filled out completely in order for you to receive proper credit. Please print clearly. Enclose a check for $15.00 payable to Dannemiller Memorial Educational Foundation. Mail to the address shown below. The Post Office will not deliver without proper postage.

Expiration Date: This credit is valid through June 30, 2001. No credit will be given after this date.

Dannemiller Memorial Educational Foundation
Attn: Contraception Report/99-40e
12500 Network Blvd., Suite 101, San Antonio, TX 78249-3302

Name _____ Degree _____

Street _____

City _____ State _____

Zip Code _____ Phone _____

Nursing License Number/State _____

Actual amount of time spent in this activity was: _____ hours _____ minutes.
(If blank, the Dannemiller Foundation assumes the participant spent 2 hours studying this material.)

Record your answers by circling the appropriate letter for each question.

11. a b c d	16. a b c d	
12. a b c d	17. a b c d	
13. a b c d	18. a b c d	
14. a b c d	19. a b c d	
15. a b c d	20. a b c d	

80% (8 correct answers) constitutes a passing grade.

Please cut this page out and send to Dannemiller with your CME fee.

Evaluation Questionnaire

Modern Oral Contraception, Section 2

1. Please rate this program with respect to:

Overall quality of material:	☐ Excellent	☐ Very Good	☐ Good	☐ Fair	☐ Poor
Content of the section:	☐ Excellent	☐ Very Good	☐ Good	☐ Fair	☐ Poor
Usefulness in your practice:	☐ Excellent	☐ Very Good	☐ Good	☐ Fair	☐ Poor
How well course objectives were met:	☐ Excellent	☐ Very Good	☐ Good	☐ Fair	☐ Poor

2. Was there commercial or promotional bias in the presentation?   ☐ Yes   ☐ No

If yes, please explain: _____

3. Additional comments: _____

_____

Your e-mail address: _____

May Dannemiller contact you regarding CME program outcomes?   ☐ Yes   ☐ No

CME Quiz Answer Form

After you have circled your answers to the questions, complete the information below and on the reverse side. This form must be filled out completely in order for you to receive proper credit. Please print clearly. Enclose a check for $15.00 payable to Dannemiller Memorial Educational Foundation. Mail to the address shown below. The Post Office will not deliver without proper postage.

Expiration Date: This credit is valid through June 30, 2001. No credit will be given after this date.

Dannemiller Memorial Educational Foundation
Attn: Contraception Report/99-40e
12500 Network Blvd., Suite 101, San Antonio, TX 78249-3302

Name _____ Degree _____

Street _____

City _____ State _____

Zip Code _____ Phone _____

Nursing License Number/State _____

Actual amount of time spent in this activity was: _____ hours _____ minutes.
(If blank, the Dannemiller Foundation assumes the participant spent 2 hours studying this material.)

Modern Oral Contraception

Record your answers by circling the appropriate letter for each question.

21. a b c d   26. a b c d

22. a b c d   27. a b c d

23. a b c d   28. a b c d

24. a b c d   29. a b c d

25. a b c d   30. a b c d

80% (8 correct answers) constitutes a passing grade.

Please cut this page out and send to Dannemiller with your CME fee.

Evaluation Questionnaire

Modern Oral Contraception, Section 3

1. Please rate this program with respect to:

Overall quality of material:	☐ Excellent	☐ Very Good	☐ Good	☐ Fair	☐ Poor
Content of the section:	☐ Excellent	☐ Very Good	☐ Good	☐ Fair	☐ Poor
Usefulness in your practice:	☐ Excellent	☐ Very Good	☐ Good	☐ Fair	☐ Poor
How well course objectives were met:	☐ Excellent	☐ Very Good	☐ Good	☐ Fair	☐ Poor

2. Was there commercial or promotional bias in the presentation?   ☐ Yes   ☐ No

   If yes, please explain: _____

3. Additional comments: _____

   _____

Your e-mail address: _____

May Dannemiller contact you regarding CME program outcomes?   ☐ Yes   ☐ No

CME Quiz Answer Form

After you have circled your answers to the questions, complete the information below and on the reverse side. This form must be filled out completely in order for you to receive proper credit. Please print clearly. Enclose a check for $15.00 payable to Dannemiller Memorial Educational Foundation. Mail to the address shown below. The Post Office will not deliver without proper postage.

Expiration Date: This credit is valid through June 30, 2001. No credit will be given after this date.

Dannemiller Memorial Educational Foundation
Attn: Contraception Report/99-40e
12500 Network Blvd., Suite 101, San Antonio, TX 78249-3302

Name _____ Degree _____

Street _____

City _____ State _____

Zip Code _____ Phone _____

Nursing License Number/State _____

Actual amount of time spent in this activity was: _____ hours _____ minutes.
(If blank, the Dannemiller Foundation assumes the participant spent 2 hours studying this material.)

Modern Oral Contraception

Record your answers by circling the appropriate letter for each question.

31. a b c d	36. a b c d
32. a b c d	37. a b c d
33. a b c d	38. a b c d
34. a b c d	39. a b c d
35. a b c d	40. a b c d

80% (8 correct answers) constitutes a passing grade.

Please cut this page out and send to Dannemiller with your CME fee.

Evaluation Questionnaire

Modern Oral Contraception, Section 4

1. Please rate this program with respect to:

Overall quality of material:	☐ Excellent	☐ Very Good	☐ Good	☐ Fair	☐ Poor
Content of the section:	☐ Excellent	☐ Very Good	☐ Good	☐ Fair	☐ Poor
Usefulness in your practice:	☐ Excellent	☐ Very Good	☐ Good	☐ Fair	☐ Poor
How well course objectives were met:	☐ Excellent	☐ Very Good	☐ Good	☐ Fair	☐ Poor

2. Was there commercial or promotional bias in the presentation?   ☐ Yes   ☐ No

   If yes, please explain: _____

3. Additional comments: _____

_____

_____

Your e-mail address: _____

May Dannemiller contact you regarding CME program outcomes?   ☐ Yes   ☐ No

Emron Quality Evaluation Form

Please use this page to send comments, suggestions, or questions to the Editorial Board of *Modern Oral Contraception*. Also, please take a moment to answer the questions below regarding quality of the book material.

Comments/Questions: _____

_____

_____

Did the material presented contain commercial or promotional bias?   ☐ Yes   ☐ No

Please rate the overall quality of the material.
☐ Excellent   ☐ Very Good   ☐ Good   ☐ Fair   ☐ Poor

Please type or print clearly.

Name _____

Title/Institution _____

Address _____

City/State/Zip _____

Modern Oral Contraception

Emron Quality Evaluation Form

Please cut out this page, place in a stamped envelope, and mail your comments to the following address:

The Contraception Report
c/o Emron
100 Campus Road
Totowa NJ 07512-9971